Studies in Disorders of Communication

General Editors:

Professor David Crystal
Honorary Professor of Linguistics, University College of North Wales,
Bangor

Professor Ruth Lesser
University of Newcastle upon Tyne

Professor Margaret Snowling
University of Newcastle upon Tyne

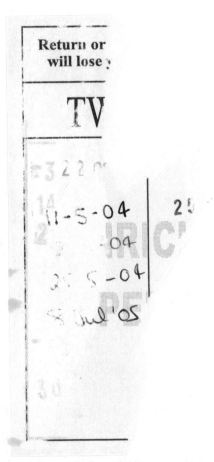

Perceptual Approaches to Communication Disorders

Edited by Sheila L. Wirz, PhD,

Centre for International Child Health, University of London

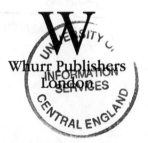

Whurr Publishers
London

First published 1995 by
Whurr Publishers Ltd
19b Compton Terrace, London N1 2UN, England

British Library Cataloguing in Publication Data
A catalogue record for this book is available from the
British Library.

ISBN 1-870332-89-X

Photoset by Stephen Cary
Printed and bound in the UK by Athenaeum Press Ltd,
Gateshead, Tyne & Wear

Foreword

As manager of a speech and language therapy service I need to know that staff are examining their clinical practices and continuing to develop their skills. The information necessary for such professional development and continuing education must be both relevant to clinical practice and easy to read.

That is why I welcome this book, written clearly and concisely by experienced and respected members of the profession. Each contributor has concentrated on a particular specialism but all have adopted a common theme: a client-centred approach to assessment rather than one driven simply by theory. We are lucky to be able to draw on such a valuable resource.

How many of us can honestly say that we know what core skills speech and language therapists possess? Yet purchasers of our therapy services have a right to know what we have to offer people with communication difficulties. We not only have to be sure in ourselves that we know what we are doing, how we are doing it, and what the outcomes are likely to be; we also have to market those skills to others.

Sheila Wirz and her contributors have defined our core skills in a way which commands respect and will enhance the confidence of speech and language therapists in the UK and abroad. We know that we have highly developed perceptual skills, both auditory and observational, which underpin the work of all clinicians, whether they work with clients with learning difficulties, childhood speech and language disorders, dysphasia, deafness or cerebral palsy. It is in the integration of these skills and their adaption to the individual personal characteristics of each client that our expertise chiefly consists. Sheila Wirz and her team have presented us with a trenchant reaffirmation of this truth and I welcome this book.

Joan Munro
Chair, College of Speech and Language Therapists

Contributors

Elizabeth Dean
Queen Margaret College, Edinburgh

Ann Edmonson
Gogarburn Hospital, Lothian Health Board, Scotland

Sally Irlam
Camden and Islington Community Health Trust, London

Margaret Leahy
School of Clinical Speech and Language, Trinity College, Dublin

Janet Mackenzie Beck
Centre for Speech Technology, University of Edinburgh

Rosemarie Morgan Barrie
National Hospital College Speech Sciences, London

Ann Parker
National Hospital College Speech Sciences, London

Christine Skinner
Queen Margaret College, Edinburgh

Sandy Winyard
Department of Rehabilitation, University of Southampton

Sheila Wirz
Centre for International Child Health, University of London

Preface

It is incumbent on any professional to remain constantly aware of those core skills which lie at the heart of their professional practice. Originally introduced through education and training they are further refined through professional experience. Within speech and language therapy many clinicians specialise in work with particular client groups and develop specialist professional skills, but the nature of their core skills is seldom explicitly defined. Yet, the ability to observe and listen critically to clients remains at their centre. Of course, the detail of observation and listening will vary within the specialism but not the clinician's basic skills.

The theme of this book is how specialist clinicians draw on their core skills as a basis for their work.

The UK is in the midst of health reforms which require all health professionals to state clearly the nature of their professional practice. It is tempting for purchasers of services to give undue priority to symptom-based specialist intervention. Speech and language therapists need to assure purchasers of their services that clients with specific communication disorders and specialist needs are best served by clinicians whose specialist intervention skills are built upon a solid core of professional skills rather than by people offering activities based on a superficial approach to the presenting symptoms.

This book draws upon the experience of clinicians in common fields of specialism. Each underlines the fact that skilled intervention is built upon a base of observation and listening to clients. The recording, transcribing and analysis of client performance is, of course, a vital part of any clinician's battery of skills, but the experienced clinician recognises above all that she is considering the performance of an individual communicator. The individual may have impaired skills but nonetheless it is a performance generated by a person and must be treated as such, not as communicative data typical of a particular disorder. The experienced clinician has the client at the centre of her practice not the disordered communicator.

This book describes first the development of assessment and then goes on to look at the perceptual skills clinicians employ in their work with six groups of clients:

- Clients with profound learning difficulties.
- Children with slow speech development.
- Deaf people.
- Aphasic people.
- People with voice disorders, and
- Communication aid users.

The book also includes a chapter on observation of self. Margaret Leahy argues that clinicians should apply their professional rigour of observation as much to their own behaviour as to the observation of clients if personal development as a clinician is to continue.

This book reaffirms the need for clinicians, in whatever work setting, to have confidence in their core skills and to demonstrate how specialist development must build upon this firm base if it is to be effective.

I thank the contributors to this book for their thoughtful discussion and varied contributions. I believe the variety of these chapters is a microcosm of the variety which attracts clinicians to speech and language therapy. I would also like to thank the many speech and language therapy students with whom I have had the privilege to work over many years. Their questions and enthusiasm helped to shape my ideas as to the nature of core skills. And, finally, may I thank the many clients with whom I have worked who have always challenged my understanding of the nature of speech and language therapy.

Sheila L. Wirz

General preface

This series focuses upon disorders of speech language and communication, bringing together the techniques of analysis, assessment and treatment which are pertinent to the area. It aims to cover cognitive, linguistic, social and education aspects of language disability, and therefore has relevance within a number of disciplines. These include speech therapy, the education of children and adults with special needs, teachers of the deaf, teachers of English as a second language and of foreign languages, and educational and clinical psychology. The research and clinical findings from these various areas can usefully inform one another and, therefore, we hope one of the main functions of this series will be to put people within one profession in touch with developments in another. Thus, it is our editorial policy to ask authors to consider the implications of their findings for professions outside their own and for fields with which they have not been primarily concerned. We hope to engender an integrated approach to theory and practice and to produce a much-needed emphasis on the description and analysis of language as such, as well as on the provision of specific techniques of therapy, remediation and rehabilitation.

Whilst it has been our aim to restrict the series to the study of language disability, its scope goes considerably beyond this. Many previously neglected topics have been included where these seem to benefit from contemporary research in linguistics, psychology, medicine, sociology, education and English studies. Each volume puts its subject matter in perspective and provides an introductory slant to its presentation. In this way we hope to provide specialised studies which can be used as texts for components of teaching courses at undergraduate and postgraduate levels, as well as material directly applicable to the needs of professional workers.

David Crystal
Ruth Lesser
Margaret Snowling

Contents

Chapter 4

Speech intelligibility and deafness: the skills of listener and speaker

Ann Parker and Sally Irlam

Chapter 5

Perceptual assessment in aphasia

Elizabeth Dean and Christine Skinner

Chapter 6

The interactive skills of young communication aid users

Sandy Winyard

Chapter 7

Chapter 8

University of Central England
Self Service receipt for items borrowed

27/11/04
04:15 pm

01762103
Item Speech and language: clinical process and practice

32040166
Due Date: 11/12/2004 23:59

Item Perceptual approaches to communication disorders

30035570
Due Date: 11/12/2004 23:59

Please retain your receipt.

Chapter 1
Assessing communication skills in diverse client groups: the role of speech and language therapy

Sheila Wirz

It is 50 years since early speech and language therapists in the UK began collaborating and sharing ideas about practice and training. During those 50 years both the knowledge base and the practice of speech and language therapy have developed immeasurably. A consequence of this development has been growth in specialism within the profession. Speech and language therapists working in the field of acquired speech and language disorders use different skills and knowledge and have a different group of working colleagues from those who work with deaf people or those working with clients with severe learning difficulties and their families*. The skills and knowledge of therapists who become aphasiologists or workers with deaf people or people with severe learning difficulties will differ but will be firmly rooted in the common ground of a speech and language therapy base.

This book reaffirms the importance of that base and stresses the value of the perceptual abilities of a speech and language therapist as the basis of therapy, regardless of specialism.

A large part of the role of a speech and language therapist is assessment. In spite of the emphasis on standardised assessment in recent years the speech and language therapist must be skilled in observing the responses of her clients in many settings and in interaction with their care-givers and others.

It is the ability of the therapist to perceive, to observe and evaluate a client's communicative strengths and weaknesses, abilities and

---

*The professions of speech pathology in North America and Australia and that of speech and language therapy in the UK have led the world in developing knowledge about communication disorder and of services for communicatively impaired people. In this volume the term 'speech and language therapist' is used to refer to the professional, because the authors are all from the UK. The term is used on the understanding that it is directly equivalent to the term 'speech pathologist' in other parts of the English-speaking world. When a pronoun is needed, the pronoun 'she' has been used to refer to the speech and language therapist and 'he' to the client.

disabilities which separates her from a teacher, a psychologist, a concerned carer, or a health worker.

It is not the purpose of this book to discuss assessment of communication disorder nor does it aim to describe exhaustively test batteries or observation procedures which could be used with different client groups. This task has been performed elsewhere, for example, by Kersner (1992) and Beech, Harding and Hilton Jones (1993). This book discusses ways in which the therapist uses her perceptual skills with different client groups.

The seven following chapters refer to different client groups and to different perceptual skills which may be used with them. These skills can be subdivided into two overlapping groups:

1. Auditory perceptual skills and the transcription skills with which to record these auditory perceptions.
2. Observation of communicative competence and changes in communicative competence with different interlocutors or different settings.

These groups of skills refer to the way in which therapists perceive client behaviour. It is equally important that therapists develop self-perceptual skills if they are to become able to perceive their own behaviour in therapy settings and be able to modify it when necessary.

The book concentrates on effective perception of communication and, in doing so, focuses on the individuality of the client, how he responds to different environments and the different people with whom he seeks to communicate. This lays a challenging burden on the therapist — not just the skills to listen accurately, to transcribe and plan an appropriate intervention programme but also to understand the fears, hopes and aspirations of her client. That is why the final chapter of the book, by Leahy, is so important. Just as the ancient Greeks believed that the beginning of all wisdom was to know oneself, so Leahy argues the central importance of self-analysis and growth for all therapists. Hers is the final chapter of the book; the other six chapters are arranged in two groups.

Chapters 2, 3 and 4 look at different aspects of perceptual skills and their transcription. Morgan Barry describes the way in which therapists can observe and record the emerging auditory skills of children; Wirz and Mackenzie Beck refer to the perception and transcription of voice quality and of disordered voice quality, and Parker and Irlam describe the way therapists can record the speech of deaf people and provide a new rating scale for intelligibility of deaf people's communication. The chapter by Parker and Irlam provides a link to the second group in that it also stresses the importance of observing speech in the context of total communicative competence.

The subsequent three chapters concentrate on the observation of communicative competence. Dean and Skinner discuss it among dysphasic people and describe a new procedure which records different components of communicative competence; Winyard describes the communicative interaction of communication aids users and suggests ways in which therapists can ascertain the communication effectiveness of the aid to the user. Finally, among this second group, Edmondson explores the ways in which therapists can observe and record the communicative attempts of people with profound hearing difficulties.

It is timely to consider the underlying core of speech and language therapy in the light of the considerable current structural upheaval within the National Health Service (NHS) in the UK. The NHS reforms in the UK have had considerable impact on all clinical services, including, of course, the delivery of speech and language therapy services. There has been a move away from services being provided at District Health Authority level to services being provided by smaller NHS Trusts or, indeed, by semi-autonomous specialist clinical directorates. Ham (1993) and Mawhinney (1993) provide a review of the progress of the NHS reforms and possible future directions for the NHS. Managers of speech and language therapy services are being asked by provider units to retain or, indeed, to increase the specialist nature of their services, whereas purchasers seek contracts for generic speech therapy services. There is a tension between the demands of purchasers for eclectic/general services, the dispersal of therapists into smaller Trusts and directorates and the increasingly informed demands by consumers and their specialist advocacy groups for specialist services. It is timely to re-examine the central core of speech and language therapy. The base upon which specialist knowledge is developed must be clearly visible to purchasers and providers if speech and language therapy is to survive and not be replaced by single-client-group specialists who have narrow technical skills but lack general knowledge and skills about communication disorders. Speech therapists' assistants have such technical skills but are neither trained to be able nor expected to undertake, the integrative functions of a therapist (TASTMS, 1993). This chapter introduces ideas about the centrality of perceptual skills in a speech and language therapist's professional practice then proceeds to give a very brief historical account of how skills of assessment and observation have developed in speech and language therapy over the past century. Secondly, it looks at some epidemiological considerations as to the size of the different client groups. Thirdly, the chapter considers the nature of service delivery and asks the question: *'Do services address the client need in terms of the individual's 'handicap' or in terms of the individual's 'disability'?'* (WHO, 1980).

Introduction

This book collects together a series of chapters relating to six commonly occurring disorders of communication, discussing: communication difficulties of deaf people; people with physical disabilities; people with severe learning difficulties; those with voice problems; those with post-traumatic aphasia; and children who fail to develop spoken language. One reason for this apparently eclectic selection is that all the authors subscribe to the view that speech and language therapists are concerned with all aspects of communication disorder, not simply with voice disorders or aphasia or communication aids. These are areas in which some speech and language therapists choose to specialise but speech and language therapy is about *people* with communication disorders, not disorders *per se*.

The second reason for this particular selection is that these chapters all concentrate on what the therapist does. It highlights not a standardised test which can be administered to clients (who may or may not have similar difficulties) but the procedures which qualified speech and language therapists use with different clients. This stance points to the centrality of communication and the communicative ability of all humans. A dysphasic adult, a stutterer, or a deaf person is somehow diminished as a communicating adult if we emphasise too much the differences amongst them as communicators. What skilled assessment should aim to do is to analyse the communicative abilities of each client. It is tautologous to assert that each client is different. Of course he is. All communicatively impaired clients are people with an individual matrix of factors which render them different from any other individual. The communicatively impaired client's communication disorder is only part of this individual matrix. It is the skill of the clinician to reveal the matrix of strengths, weaknesses, opportunities and closed doors which is available to a specific client.

The third reason for this collection of eight chapters is to reassert the importance of a therapist's own perceptions. Speech and language therapists' training in the UK (and elsewhere) is still firmly rooted in phonetics training. In Chapter 4, Parker and Irlam refer to 'the perceptual filtering effect of the assessor's own particular linguistic system'. Experienced speech and language therapists maintain their perceptual skills and have confidence in their observation skills.

Assessment falls into two categories: descriptive and prescriptive. Descriptive assessment describes, often in very great detail, the communicative behaviour of an individual — both the communicative strategies and the communicative structures used. Prescriptive assessment aims to identify communicative differences and to pinpoint how these could be remediated. The chapters of this book concentrate on perceptual assessment: those procedures which call upon clinicians' skills without dependence upon standardised assessment or instrumental measurements. Lesser and Milroy (1987) caution that perceptual assessment should not be too eclectic if it is to be effective. One of the purposes of this book is to emphasise that focused perceptual assessment can be a highly effective investigative tool

Historical overview

Speech and language therapy as a discipline has a long pre-history and a well documented recent history over the past 50 years. The developments in our understanding of disorders of communication and how to alleviate their impact has increased greatly since the 1940s. It is not simply chauvinist to assert that this development has been most apparent in the English-speaking world. This book, which looks at the role of perceptual assessment in speech and language therapy, must first consider the emerging skills of our predecessors.

Speech and language therapy developed as a discipline from its roots in medicine, especially psychiatry, neurology, ENT, and phonetics, with smaller roots in education and 'speech training', and later branch roots from psychology and linguistics. Speech and language therapy followed the research traditions of these established disciplines, especially those of medicine, psychology and linguistics, in order to achieve credibility within them.

In the early part of this century speech and language therapists fell broadly into two groups: those concerned with the mechanics of speech and those who concentrated on speakers' psychological behaviour. The first group included those who embraced the new knowledge derived from phonetics. Phoneticians, such as Aitken (1910), developed descriptions of disordered speech and voice in addition to increasingly sophisticated descriptions of the speech process. These descriptive tools were used to describe disordered speech. Secondly, there were those who concentrated more on the psychological behaviour of 'speech disordered' people (Fremel and Froeschells, 1914). Early clinicians working in or in association with these areas developed their listening skills in the tradition of early phoneticians. These early speech and language therapists used many convoluted threads to spin a web of lateral stigmatisms, interdental stigmatisms, lisping, lalling, rhotacisms and others, to attract and sustain the interest of their early phonetician colleagues (Stein, 1942).

Those early therapists who worked with disordered voices (notably with singers) in the early part of this century also developed their listening skills. Early voice therapists integrated knowledge from at least two very different disciplines, anatomy and phonetics, with skills from singing and/or voice production. This integration of knowledge has been vital in the emergence of speech and language therapy as an independent speciality during the twentieth century. The developing confidence of researchers and practitioners to take from the knowledge base of other disciplines without being restricted by their limitations has marked the maturity of speech and language therapy.

Mention, too, must be made of those early practitioners who worked with neurologists to investigate and ameliorate the communication difficulties of young men injured during the First World War. The comparatively discrete damage of gunshot wounds to young, fit men enabled investigators to move the study of acquired speech and language disorders forward (Weisenburg and McBride, 1926).

Later, two of the most influential early speech and language therapists, Morley (1957) in the UK and Templin (1957) in the USA, collected data about children who exhibited communication disorders in a way which their medical paediatric colleagues recognised and approved. These investigations prepared the ground for epidemiological incidence and prevalence studies of communication disorder in children but are firmly rooted in the categories of the medical model, where 'causative factors' are often used to describe categories. The methodology of these early group data studies may have been rooted in medical practice, but the impact on speech and language therapy was to highlight the need to differentiate between developmentally delayed and disordered communication in children. Before their work little heed was paid to this important difference.

One of the pitfalls into which early 'speech' or 'articulation' assessment fell was that there was no attempt to define error in developmental terms. Errors were simply seen as non-adult forms. The work of Morley (1957) laid the foundations for assessments which began to separate delayed from disordered speech in children with production difficulties.

As the body of knowledge about human communication, communication disorder and progress of disorder developed, assessment of communicatively impaired people moved first from being diagnosis centred towards assessments based on the norms of group data. It became common for assessments of child language, which were based on norms, to express their scores in terms of 'language age' or 'articulation age' (e.g. Anthony et al., 1971), and for assessments of adults with acquired disorders to express these difficulties in terms of 'normative data' (e.g. Schuell, 1965). With this emphasis both on milestones and on grouped data there emerged a series of assessments which looked at deficits; the ways in which the person with a communication disorder failed.

Commonly, the aim of such assessments was to determine how an individual's communicative behaviour compared with that of his peers. Such comparative assessments made use of developmental milestones derived from studies of the acquisition of a particular skill by groups of children, or normative data derived from standardisation procedures where the responses of groups of healthy people to tasks are recorded and used as a baseline for comparison. These standardised assessment procedures took little account of the fact that the client may not want to jump through the 'communicative hoops' of the assessment. Communication perhaps more than any other behaviour has, as a vital prerequisite, the *need* to communicate. If that *need* is absent one must ask how representative the resulting behaviour really is.

The 1960s and 1970s saw much research into communication disorder following the group study approaches used by contemporary psychologists and medical physicians (Darley, Aronson and Brown, 1975). At the same time certain communication disorders were examined by use of new analyses from branches of linguistics. In the 1960s linguistics was an emerging discipline which was to develop concepts which greatly enhanced speech and language therapy, notably the development of new assessments. Some linguists became increasingly interested in communication disorder, especially language disorders. This interest had a limited effect on contemporary standardised language assessments (Reynell, 1969) but more important was the impact which linguists had upon assessment practice. The *Language Analysis Remediation and Screening Procedure* (LARSP) (Crystal et al., 1976) is a classic example of a procedure which used linguistic principles to affect therapists' assessment behaviour. It was procedures such as LARSP which were influential in moving clinical assessment of communication disorder away from standardised tests to standard procedures. A fuller account of changing practice in assessment in speech and language therapy is included in Eldredge (1968) and Wirz (1993).

Three especially interesting directions for speech and language therapy emerged from linguistics and psychology in the late 1960s. The impact of these three areas: pragmatic theory; instrumental innovation; and cognitive psychology, persists today. First, the growth in pragmatic theory led to greater understanding of the use which people make of communication. The impact of linguistic principles upon the assessment of language structures was referred to above. Similarly, the impact of pragmatic theory affected assessment practice at this time. Sarno (1969) suggested that assessment of dysphasic clients could be enhanced by the use of standard procedures to determine clients' communicative abilities in real situations.

Second, instrumental innovations led to changes in both assessments and in augmentative communication aids. This is expanded upon by Winyard in Chapter 6.

Third, there was the developing study of cognitive psychology and the application which this had to our understanding of communication breakdown. The impact of cognitive psychology upon speech and language therapy demanded a reappraisal of our understanding and management of language disorder, both developmental and acquired. Not only has this change affected assessment and management procedures but it has also given speech and language therapy increased confidence to move away from dependence on large group studies to prove efficacy. The growth of the single-case-study design as an investigative approach to the study of communication disorder, as well as being used as an assessment tool for individuals, has been especially evident since the mid-1980s (Byng and Coltheart, 1986; Pring, 1986). Cognitive psychology has given speech and language therapy the credibility of assessment based on a problem-solving approach either instead of or in conjunction with standardised assessments.

The importance of this position in the developing confidence of speech pathology as an independent discipline should not be underestimated. Investigations and observational routines were in danger of concentrating on the analysis of the symptoms of communication disorder to the exclusion of the inter-relationships behind these symptoms. The inter-relationships of symptoms is at the heart of understanding communication breakdown and a skilled therapist has the ability to synthesise specific areas of analysis.

Early assessment procedures measured differences in response between impaired and non-impaired communicators. More recently, in the 1980s, assessment has moved from concentrating on responses to an examination of the processes involved in communication. Thus, 20 years ago, for example, the aim of a speech assessment was to show how the target articulatory behaviour of a speaker differed from the norm. For example, Fisher and Logeman (1971) scored percentage correct in terms of targets and more specifically percentage correct in terms of 'place', 'manner' or 'voicing' of the target. The aim of recent speech assessment is likely to be an examination of the phonological process underpinning that articulatory behaviour. Grunwell (1985) was instrumental in the move from describing the symptoms of communicative differences to examining communicative processes. Parker and Irlam, below, expand upon the importance of understanding phonological processes, not errors, if the therapist is to identify contributory components of unintelligibility. This emphasis on communication processes and damage to processes is helpful in explaining both group and individual differences.

It is an oversimplification to suggest that there are two forms of client assessment, micro-assessment and macro-assessment, but such a simplification provides a useful working model. On the one hand, 'micro investigations' help to build up a picture of a client's breakdown (or poor development) of a single aspect of communication. For example, such investigations might concentrate on single-word processing of spoken or read material, production of single words in spoken or written forms, processing of input by colour, size, semantic category, phonemic form, etc. etc. On the other hand, 'macro investigations' are those which by selective choice from these same procedures use several investigations to inform the clinician about a range of the client's processing abilities and, within the context of case history information, enhance remedial planning.

The skill for the practising clinician is to select those procedures appropriate to the individual client. Within this skilful selection there is a danger that the clinician might assess in ever-decreasing circles of investigative detail. The danger is that such detail may not inform the rehabilitative plan.

The Renaissance saw a flowering of art and science. The art remains to delight us today, but how often do we look to the scientific heritage of that period to reaffirm our understanding of order. Early Renaissance thinkers believed that all behaviour could be explained by the relationships between physical, metaphysical and religious laws; that all behaviour contributed to the unity of the universe. Later Renaissance saw a movement away from this three-fold explanation of unity, with greater emphasis on scientific explanation. We are now amused by the complex diagrams, mathematical workings and explanations of Kepler* and others in their attempts to explain universality, but at the end of the twentieth century is speech pathology in danger of misusing scientific enquiry, of behaving like Kepler and trying to discover unity where none may exist? It is necessary in a field as small (in relative terms) as that of communication disorders to ensure that we use the investigative tools appropriately. There is a danger of speech and language therapists hitching their investigative credibility to the traditions of medicine, psychology and the high altar of statistics at times when such practice can endanger the search for explanations of communication disorder.

Epidemiological considerations

To say that the size of the communicatively impaired population is relatively small is both accurate and provocative. It is difficult to determine the size of this population. The Royal Commission chaired by Randolph Quirk (Quirk, 1972) aimed to determine the numbers of speech and language therapists required to provide a speech therapy service for the NHS in the UK. It was not the primary aim of the Commission to determine the size of the communicatively impaired population. Perforce they did, of course, in their deliberations give a clearer picture of the size of this population in England and Wales. The Commission estimated that around 0.6% of the population had a communication disorder of such severity as to need the help of a speech and language therapist.

In the 20 years since the publication of the Quirk Report, speech and language services have developed into areas of service which were

*Johann Kepler (1571–1630), German astronomer; his First and Second Laws in *Astronoma Nova* (1609) formed the groundwork of Newton's discoveries.

almost unknown in the 1960s and 1970s. Specialist speech and language therapy with deaf people, with people with severe learning difficulties and with communication aids users were almost unknown 20 years ago, apart from a few individual enthusiastic pioneers working in these fields in considerable isolation. Services such as these are now regularly provided alongside the mainstay services of speech and language therapy for children and for adults with acquired disorders. These 'mainstay services' which were the two parts of speech and language therapy unified after the recommendations of the Quirk Report have also become increasingly specialist over these 20 years.

With the NHS reforms of the early 1990s there has been a move from profession-led to client-led services. It is no longer sufficient justification to have a professional interest in developing new services (if indeed it ever should have been) for unserved client need. Purchasing authorities will have to be convinced of the need for such services before they will place contracts to enable new developments.

Studies by Enderby and Phillips (1986) and Enderby and Davies (1989) have more recently attempted to define the size of the communicatively impaired population in the UK. They estimate that 2.3 million people (or 4.2% of the population) have a communication disorder and that around 1.5% of the total population had a disorder of sufficient severity to merit the help of a speech therapist, an estimate double that of Quirk. In the second study, Enderby chose not to provide a total picture of incidence but rather to show incidence of communication problems in subpopulations, e.g. of learning disordered people, head injured people, etc.

In a service such as speech and language therapy where the total potential client population is small, estimates vary from 0.6% of the population (Quirk, 1972) to 1.5% (Enderby and Phillips, 1986); the subgroups of communicatively impaired clients with different communication problems will perforce be even smaller. The subsequent six chapters of this book reflect, in the main, the larger groups of communicatively impaired people. Enderby and Phillips (1986) suggest prevalence rates of communication disorder related to:

• Learning disorders of 13.75%.
• Childhood speech and language difficulties of 5.5%.
• Acquired language difficulties after cardiovascular accident of 1.5%.
• Deafness 1.2%.
• Cerebral palsy of 1.1%.

The subsequent chapters of this book address the question of how best to determine the communication needs of clients within these populations.

What do speech and language therapy services address?

This may seem at first reading to be an obvious question. Speech and language therapy services address the needs of communicatively impaired clients. The thesis of this book is that this is not always the case. Sometimes therapy is directed at the disorder not the person with the communication disorder; at the therapist's perception of what is helpful, not at the client's or carer's perceived needs. The chapters of this book all emphasise the need to observe the client, for the therapist to use her eyes and ears to see beyond the communication disorder and encompass a wider perception of the client's need. Only thus can speech and language therapy be truly effective for the client.

There has been much discussion from a number of sources as to the scientific nature of speech pathology (Ringel, Trachtman and Prutting, 1984; Eastwood, 1988). It is important in an introductory chapter of this volume to take cognisance of the effect which this debate has upon assessment practice. In attempts to understand communication disorder more fully, researchers have used research techniques proven in other fields. Too great an emphasis on empirical evidence to determine ever-decreasing circles of detail regarding specific disorders can distort the understanding of the phenomenon being examined. Bench (1991) reminds us that scientific method does not equate with empirical study and that observational techniques in a field as multifaceted as human communication are often a more appropriate investigative tool. There is a danger that practitioners forget that whichever aspect of communication disorder is being investigated it is the disturbance of human communication which is central and remains as the backdrop to specific investigations of detail.

The World Health Organization's *Classification of Impairments, Disability and Handicap* (WHO, 1980) offers a different dimension to this potential difficulty for speech and language therapy. This classification defines:

- Impairment as 'abnormalities of body, structure, appearance, organ or system function resulting from any cause'.
- Disability as 'the consequences of the impairment in terms of functional performance and activity'.
- Handicap as 'the disadvantages experienced by the individual as a result of the impairments and disabilities' (WHO, 1980, pp. 14–16).

This distinction of impairment, disability and handicap throws into sharp focus the differences between researchers who seek explanation for the impairment (or 'system (dys)function (WHO, 1980, p. 14)) and the clinician who seeks assessment tools for the disability (or 'consequences of the impairment in terms of the functional performance and activity by the individual' (WHO, 1980, p. 15)). There is a danger that researchers who use empirical methodologies appropriately in the pursuit of explanations about communication disorder (or 'impairment') unintentionally mislead practitioners to employ similar methodologies in their assessment practice of 'disability'. Skilled clinicians are aware of this distinction and use information from researchers' investigations of impairment to inform their clinical practice where they will be considering disabilities.

Types of assessment

The assessment tools available to clinicians can be classified in a number of ways. One way is to divide investigative tools into three groups:

1. Inventories of skills or inventories of deficits.
2. 'Test' batteries which examine (or purport to examine) assets or those which examine weaknesses.
3. Assessment procedures which attempt to examine all the communication skills of a client to those which examine specific skills.

A further dichotomy exists between those assessments which can be described as 'client-centred', evaluating the strengths and/or weaknesses of a particular client, and those which can be described as 'disorder-centred', concentrating as they do on the common features of a particular disorder.

The rich choice available to therapists is both daunting and exciting. The therapist must determine from a matrix of possibilities which type of assessment is suitable for her client:

- An inventory of assets or one of deficits.
- A test battery designed to determine levels of achievement or those of failure.
- A procedure with eclectic or specific application.
- A procedure which examines behaviours or processes.
- A procedure designed for all media of communication or only some.

The choice of assessment procedure is crucial if the total needs of the communicatively impaired client are to be assessed. An assessment of most disordered communication will include an assessment of communicative strategies of the close family with the client. The communicative behaviour of the family is seen by the authors in this book to be of equal importance with that of the client himself in a full assessment preceding any intervention. The primary goal of the assessment of communication disorders is to identify the difficulties for the client exhibiting communication disorder and to determine how these impact on the client's life. If therapists lose sight of this primary goal, they are no longer speech and language therapists but rather applied linguists, cognitive psychologists, special educators, phoniatrists or other.

All the chapters in this book stress that assessment of all the client groups must be carried out in the context of full information about the client, his communicative needs, his family circumstances and communicative skills. Without detailed information about the client and his needs, any assessment becomes the analysis of data rather than the assessment of the communication in an individual. One of the characteristics of therapists is that they consider these needs and are not wooed into thinking of clients as data-producing mechanisms. It is the complexity of the communication process and the idiosyncrasies of each client which challenge the clinician both in assessment and in interpreting the findings in each assessment that is undertaken.

This rich variety offers the speech and language therapist a challenge. She must describe whether the assessment is undertaken as a measurement tool to establish a baseline for therapy; as an investigatory procedure leading to a diagnosis of need; as an evaluation of the efficacy of intervention; or as a screening procedure to pinpoint areas for further investigations. With whichever client group, using whatever media of communication and measurement, the value of a therapist to a client with disordered communication will only be as good as the assessment which precedes the planning of an intervention programme and the assessments which evaluate efficacy throughout the implementation of that programme.

Four of the chapters in this volume concentrate upon the way in which the clinician assesses the communicative skills of clients rather than their specific deficits or differences in communicative behaviour.

In Chapter 4, the assessment of the communication skills of severely and profoundly deaf people is an area where speech therapists have developed tools to assess communication by use of different media of communication. Speech and language therapists working with this client group need to undertake assessments in both British Sign Language (BSL) and Sign Supported English (SSE) as well as in spoken English in an attempt to ascertain the language and communication skills of their clients. Parker and Irlam demonstrate how important it is for the therapist to have good communication skills and experience of deaf speech if they are satisfactorily to attempt an assessment of a deaf person's intelligibility.

In dysphasia assessment, too, therapists seek information in their assessments from a range of different media. In Chapter 5, Dean and Skinner describe how all aspects of communication must be described if a full picture of the abilities and needs of a dysphasic person is to be established. They assert that to emphasise the difficulties which a dysphasic person has is only a small part of a full assessment and stress the need for flexibility by therapists.

With advances in computer technology and speech synthesis a small but significant group of disabled people have come to depend on computer-aided communication. In Chapter 6, Winyard describes the assessment which must precede the choice of aid; the selection of an appropriate interface by which the disabled person can use the aid; and the acceptability of the aid to the client and his family. She also demonstrates that it is not only the client who must be familiarised with the aid and helped to explore its use but emphasises that the family, too, will not use the communicative potential of aided communication without help.

In Chapter 7, Edmonson also stresses that the communicative skills of the carers and supporters of people with profound intellectual disabilities are vital if the disabled person is to use his communicative abilities to maximum potential. In her chapter, Edmunson emphasises the need for sensitivity to rudimentary communicative behaviours. She further stresses awareness of the fact that assessment of the communicative skills of this client group is a long-term process with evidence being accumulated over a period of time.

Two chapters concentrate on the perceptual assessment of a specific aspect of communication: Morgan Barry on the auditory perceptual skills of children in Chapter 2, and Wirz and Mackenzie Beck on speakers' voice quality in Chapter 3. Morgan Barry concentrates upon the components of auditory skills in children and emphasises the need to be aware of the way in which these components may develop at different rates in different children. She publishes for the first time a work-in-progress version of her *Auditory Skills Battery* which offers an assessment procedure to determine a child's auditory attention, auditory dissemination, and auditory memory.

Wirz and Mackenzie Beck describe the *Vocal Profiles Analysis Scheme*, a perceptual assessment of voice quality. Voice quality is the aspect of communication which pervades all communicative disabilities and in this chapter Wirz and Mackenzie Beck show how a perceptual scheme can be used to describe voice quality objectively. This scheme has been widely taught through workshops but has not been published in this definitive form before.

The three chapters by Morgan Barry, Wirz and Mackenzie Beck, and Parker and Irlam also stress the need for good replicable transcription skills if speech and language therapists are to record accurately their auditory perceptions of differing aspects of the client's vocal output. In contrast, Leahy concentrates not upon the perceptual assessment of clients but on the need for clinicians to examine and understand their own communicative skills. She demonstrates that for clinicians to be truly effective they must assess not only the communicative skills of the clients and their interlocutors but also develop personal awareness of their own therapeutic communicative skills.

The chapters all emphasise the need for therapists to use observational skills. The way in which these can be organised for different client groups is important but the common need for observations to be both reflective and exploratory is reiterated in all the chapters. A good practising speech and language therapist is not in a rut of established observational practice, blindly following administrative routines. She is a person who is aware of the need to use these observational skills creatively with each client. Only thus can observations be explorative and reflective of the abilities of the client and usefully inform remedial planning.

References

Aitken, W.A. (1910) *The Voice*. London: Longman

Anthony, A., Ingram, T., McIssac, A. and Boyle, D. (1971) *Edinburgh Articulation Test*. Edinburgh: Livingstone

Beech, J., Harding, L. and Hilton Jones, D. (eds) (1993) *Assessment in Speech and Language*. London: Routledge–NFER

Bench, R.J. (1991) Paradigms, methods and the epistemology of speech pathology: some comments on Eastwood. *British Journal of Disorders of Communication*, 26, 235–242

Byng, S. and Coltheart, M. (1986) Aphasia therapy research requirements. In: Ajelmquist, E. and Nilsson, L. (eds) *Communication and Handicap*. Holland: Elsevier

Crystal, D., Fletcher, P. and Garman, M. (1976) *The Grammatical Analysis of Language Disability*. London: Whurr

Darley, F.L., Aronson, A.E. and Brown, J. (1975) *Motor Speech Disorders*. Philadelphia: Saunders

Eastwood, J. (1988) Qualitative research: an additional research methodology for speech pathology? *British Journal of Disorders of Communication*, 23, 171–184

Eldredge, M. (1968) *A History of the Treatment of Speech Disorders*. Edinburgh: Livingstone

Enderby, P. and Davies, P. (1989) Communication disorders: planning a service to meet the needs. *British Journal of Disorders of Communication*, 24, 301–331

Enderby, P. and Phillips, R. (1986) Speech, language handicaps: towards knowing the size of the problems. *British Journal of Disorders of Communication*, 21, 151–165

Fisher, H.B. and Logeman, J.A. (1971) *Test of Articulatory Competence*. Boston: Houghton Mifflin

Fremel, F. and Froeschells, E. (1914) Gohor und Sprach. *Arch. Exp. and Klin. Phon.*

Goodglass, H. and Kaplan, E. (1972) *The Assessment of Aphasia and Related Disorders*. Philadelphia: Lea and Febiger

Grunwell, P. (1985) *The Phonological Assessment of Child Speech (PACS)*. Windsor: NFER-Nelson

Ham, C. (1993) *The New Natural Health Service, Organisation and Management*. Oxford: Radcliffe Medical Press

Kersner, M. (1992) *Tests in Voice, Speech and Language*. London: Whurr

Lesser, R. and Milroy L. (1987) Two frontiers in aphasia therapy. *Bulletin of the College of Speech Therapists*, **420**, 1–4

Mawhinney (1993) *Purchasing for Health: A Framework for Action*. Leeds: NHS Executive

Morley, M. (1957) *Disorders of Speech in Childhood*. Edinburgh: Livingstone

Pring, T.R. (1986) Evaluating the effects of speech therapy for aphasics: developing a single case methodology. *British Journal of Disorders of Communication*, **21**, 1, 103–116

Quirk, R. (1972) *Speech Therapy Services*. London: HMSO

Reynell, J. (1986) *The Reynell Language Development Scales*. Windsor: NFER-Nelson

Ringel, R., Trachtman, L. and Prutting, C. (1984) The science in human communication sciences. *ASHA*, **26**. 33–37

Sarno, M.T. (1969) *The Functional Communication Profile: New York Institute of Rehabilitative Medicine*. New York: University Medical Center

Schuell, M. (1965) *The Minnesota Test for Differential Diagnosis of Aphasia*. Minneapolis: University of Minnesota Press

Stein, L. (1942) *Speech and Voice – Their Evolution, Pathology and Therapy*. London: Methuen

TASTMS. (1993) *Core Curriculum for Speech and Language Therapists' Assistants*. Ponteland Stass

Templin, M. (1957) *Certain Language Skills in Children*. Minneapolis: University of Minnesota Press

WHO (1980) *The World Health Organization: Classification of Impairments, Disability and Handicap*. Geneva: WHO

Wirz, S. (1993) Introduction to assessment. In: Beech, J., Harding, L. and Hilton Jones, D. (eds) *Assessment in Speech and Language Therapy*. London: Routledge

Wirz, S., Dean, E.C. and Benham, F. (1989) Towards an understanding of communicative effectiveness in aphasia. Institute of Neurology Research Report LOCR No. 1022. London: University of London

Chapter 2
Observing and assessing auditory skills in children

Rosemarie Morgan Barrie

Auditory perception is a complex process which involves a number of skill areas. These skills can be represented as an interconnected chain of abilities, each of which is related to and dependent on the other, and which enable the hearer to detect sound as a sensory event at one end of the chain and to make sense of it as a cognitive event at the other. Thus, the set of processes involves a sensory modality with a number of perceptual–cognitive skills. The clinician needs to understand this chain of abilities and to be aware that there are differential developmental aspects to its components. There are four principal components of this complex process:

1. *Auditory acuity*, the first link in the chain, is the sensory response to sound related to a fully functioning hearing mechanism. The subsequent skills are all, to a greater or lesser extent, dependent on this ability.
2. *Auditory attention* follows from the sound pick-up ability and involves, first, an alerting to sound, followed by a mental registration of the importance (salience) of the sound to the listener. Discrimination and memory are therefore linked to this ability in that the individual will selectively screen sounds against past experience to determine levels of 'newness', non-recognition or importance to the present situation, and decide whether they deserve continuing attention and responsive action, or attention switch-off. Many factors influence auditory attention: changes in sound in the environment — of intensity, pitch or quality; the beginning of a new sound or cessation of an old one; the individual's mental set, physical state, interest and motivation.
3. *Auditory discrimination* may be defined as the ability to distinguish different properties of sounds. To the speech clinician this is the skill which helps a listener to determine the differences between the speech sounds that signal meaning changes in language. In this

sense, therefore, it is linguistically dependent. But as a general auditory skill, discrimination is used to distinguish the different qualities of environmental and natural sounds, for example: different notes in a piece of music, or the qualities of different musical instruments; the sound of a car engine in different gears; changes in mechanical sounds; different animal noises and birdsongs. Discriminatory ability, therefore, distinguishes between small differences in sounds that belong to the same type or category. Memory is also involved in that changes in the features or quality of the sounds are matched against previous awareness, knowledge, experience and expectation.

4. *Auditory memory* is the ability to retain awareness of sound in its absence and, therefore, to recognise, match and contrast one sound against another. What is retained in memory is closely linked with acuity and discrimination. But memory for speech also carries a time-sequential component and a strong semantic link. Speech sounds are serially ordered in specific sequences across syllables, words, phrases and sentences, with associated stress and intonation patterns marking out chunks of sound which are probably retained as semantic schematic wholes (Baddele, 1986).

The rationale for this division of auditory perceptual ability into related skill areas is both experimental and clinical. Aram and Nation (1982) identify a series of studies from both clinical and experimental viewpoints through the 1960s and 1970s, and subsequently describe five 'auditory operations':

- Attention.
- Rate.
- Discrimination.
- Memory.
- Sequencing.

Borden and Harris (1980) and Daniloff, Schuckers and Feth (1980) provide acoustic–physiological correlates for speech sound perception incorporating similar subcomponents. Clinical experience has both led to, and followed from, experimental studies. Speech and language therapists, working with children (and adults) with phonetic, phonological and language processing disorders have identified the skill areas of auditory attention, auditory discrimination, and auditory memory as being potential contributory factors to these disorders, and have found that focusing therapy on these factors has brought about changes in speech-production ability. It should be remembered that there is an overlapping developmental element between these aspects in that auditory attention begins to develop in children before (and later alongside) phonological discrimination which, in turn, precedes then runs concurrently with the development of auditory memory.

The exact nature of the relationship between speech–language perception and production, albeit much discussed, has not yet been resolved (Locke, 1980; Monnin, 1984; Morgan, 1984; Winitz, 1984). Nevertheless, there remains a strongly held clinical belief, partly borne out by research studies (Locke, 1980) that such a relationship exists. This is upheld by clinicians carrying out evaluations, assessments and tests, and finding that a number of children presenting with speech and language disorders of various kinds perform less well than their normal speaking peers in these auditory skill areas (Tallal and Stark, 1980; Wilcox, Daniloff and Ali, 1984; Morgan Barry, 1988).

However, it should be stressed that the assignment of skill area labels in the whole area of auditory perception varies according to the bias of different authors. As mentioned above, auditory attention is a prerequisite for both discrimination and memory; auditory memory is necessary for discrimination, whereas discrimination plays its part in attention by providing the means to appreciate novelty and interest in auditory stimuli. The ability to make sense of such stimuli is essential to maintain attention, make discriminations and compare current sounds with previous ones. Zubrick (1984) considers the relationship between attentional listening skills and verbal comprehension, and describes the following reasons for good versus poor (speech) listening ability:

- Appropriate versus inappropriate language level.
- Interest versus disinterest of listener.
- Much versus little pre-knowledge of content.
- Few versus many distractions from other sensory inputs.
- Novelty versus familiarity (a moderate level of each is needed for good listening).
- Importance versus unimportance of material.
- Maturity versus immaturity of general attention control.

The clinician must consider the implications of these when carrying out assessments of her own devising and, in particular, when planning therapy for listening and comprehension skills. Other professionals working with a child who has been found to have problems in these areas also need to be alerted to the above factors.

It may be important at this point to consider the perception of speech sounds in children with phonological and language disorders. A review of some of the questions posed in the literature concerning auditory skill assessments and their relationship to perceptual and production abilities is now presented.

Beginning with children who present with speech–language problems at phonological level, we can ask six questions:

1. What do these children perceive to be happening (auditorily) in the world around them?

2. How do they perceive adult speech?
3. How do they perceive their own speech?
4. Is there a mismatch between the two? If so
5. How do they attempt to resolve it?
6. What is going on in the child's head?

Elbert and Geirut (1986) pose the problem that it is difficult to determine the level of a child's competence in the sound system when competence refers to covert knowledge rather than overt production. Hewlett (1990; Figure 1) proposed the two-lexicon theory and model, based on empirical evidence provided by Schwartz and Leonard 1982, in which the child gains awareness of phonological contrasts from perception of adult speech and stores these in the input lexicon, and in parallel has phonological representations based on his own articulatory ability stored in the output lexicon. Realisation rules map the perceptual representations on to articulatory representations. The model provides theoretical answers to some of the questions posed above in that it suggests that where the child cannot say what he knows, phonologically speaking, he says what he can according to the realisation rules operating at that moment of articulatory development.

However, children with speech–language problems pose a number of further questions, which Locke (1980) summarises as follows:

• Are these children aware of different phonetic targets?
• Do they know their forms are not the adult forms?
• Because perception processes can only be inferred from behavioural responses, how do we know what the children are responding to?

Locke (1980a) reviews various types of auditory and perceptual assessments (these will be discussed below under the skill headings already outlined) and also proposes the *Speech Production-Perception Task* (Locke, 1980b), in which the children's own mispronunciations are given back in a comparison test with both the correct realisation and an alternative incorrect production. Many (but not all) children rejected their own productions. Why?

• Because they knew that was not how the adult ought to say the word?
• Because the adult's mispronunciation did not match their perception of how they said the word?
• Because they were unaware of the difference between their word and the adult target?

It may be put forward that children's perceptions of their own productions depend on a number of feedback processes, including kinaesthetic and proprioceptive awareness and sub-phonemic cueing, which influence the way they cope with differences between input and output lexicons. According to Locke (1980):

... the normally hearing child perceives differentially the sounds he produces distinctively, and may or may not, evidence discrimination of the sounds he collapses in production (p. 465).

The speech–language therapist, in her task of initial delineation of contributory aetiological factors for an individual child, has to balance a number of different possibilities:

- That the child has impaired articulation due to a motor production problem.
- That the child has impaired perceptual ability due to a sensory\perceptual problem.
- That the child has a phonological problem due to a cognitive–linguistic processing problem.
- That the child has a reluctance to communicate due to emotional problems.

Clinical experience proposes that these factors are not mutually exclusive; indeed, to some extent may always co-exist and overlap. (See the case study of Tommy below).

The auditory skills under discussion relate mainly to the second and third of the above possibilities, and will be the focus of the remainder of this chapter. The clinician needs to consider auditory skills in relation to a number of aspects:

- Our present understanding of the relationship of each of the skills outlined above to speech and language production and cognitive development in children.
- Means of assessment of these abilities — formal and informal, objective and perceptual, standardised and non-standardised.
- The evaluation of these methods to each other and to the outcome of therapy.

Therapy skills

The skill areas discussed here will be those of auditory attention, discrimination and memory. The assessment of auditory acuity does not fall within the brief of this chapter. Appendix I presents a pre-publication version of a new auditory skills assessment battery which aims to cover various cognitive aspects of perception, but which is still in an experimental design stage.

Auditory attention

According to Murphy (1972) auditory attention is a prerequisite for the following aspects of perceptual and cognitive development:

- Auditory response and discrimination.
- Auditory concept relating to decoding and encoding.
- Vocabulary acquisition and memory processes.
- Social readiness and contact.
- Self-monitoring.

There are two problems relating to the assessment of auditory attention; the first is that there is always an element of choice involved. A listener may decide whether or not to attend to a sound. Indeed, it is necessary to be selective in our listening, and this is idiosyncratic and related to emotional needs and cognitive associations (Murphy, 1972). The child who cannot control sensory selectivity has serious problems of attentional learning and behavioural response and may present as hyperactive, impulsive and with severe learning difficulties. Selectivity as a conscious decision also applies to the response given to a sound. However, 'the processes of perception are inescapably private' (Locke, 1980, p. 433) and an individual may give no indication of having heard a sound or be paying attention to it. A child in class may be giving every indication (by exhibiting distracter behaviour) of *not* paying attention to the teacher's words but when questioned will reproduce those words perfectly, often to his own surprise and the teacher's disbelief. In contrast, a student may give every appearance of paying close attention to a lecture, but may be thinking of something completely different.

The listener's choice of what and how much he should attend to depends on various factors, including:

- Ability to hear well enough (acuity).
- Interest and motivation.
- Importance and meaning of the sound for the individual.
- General well-being.

In order to assess auditory attention, especially in a child, the clinician's skills in assessment are critical in that she needs to determine a measure of voluntary conditioning from the child and be alert to the responses made according to pre-agreed behaviours.

The second problem relating to the assessment of auditory attention concerns the relationship between attention as a *listening* and as a *general* ability. The latter is concerned with factors, such as the amount of time and concentration an individual spends on one particular activity, general interest and motivation, and carrying a task to completion. Cooper, Moodley and Reynell (1978) have charted the development of attention in children and provided guidelines for the recognition of normal stages of development. Cooke and Williams (1985) provide ideas and activities for promoting and encouraging both general attentional and listening skills. They outline a number of factors which may contribute to poor attention in young children, and add 'the child's level of attention and the exact nature of the problem must be accurately assessed' (Cooke and Williams, 1985, p. 6).

But accurate assessment involves not only a picture of what the child *does* do but also what he *can* do ('ordinary versus optimal performance' (Jenkins, 1980)) and, as a means of comparison, what the child's peers can do also.

Skills which are not specifically task-performance related are difficult to score numerically and, therefore, to test objectively; auditory attention falls into this category. The speech and language clinician has therefore to rely on her observation skills, but these can be formalised to provide a reasonably clear picture of a child's abilities. For example, the sensory integration link between auditory and visual stimuli can be observed as follows:

- Does the child turn accurately and consistently toward a sound source, or have problems locating its direction?
- How frequently, and under what circumstances does the response occur, or not occur?
- Is this ability affected by amount and type of ongoing accompanying environmental noise?

There are also a number of general behaviours which, in the preschool child, act as pointers toward poor auditory attention. These are:

- Few or slow responses to auditory cues, in particular strongly salient ones, such as calling the child's name.
- Fidgeting during specific listening activities.
- A high level of physical activity.
- Alternatively, quietness, lethargy and reluctance to take part in group games.

There are a number of specific activities which can be used as assessments of auditory attention (see also ideas for listening games in Cooke and Williams, 1985); most clinicians will be familiar with these:

- Introducing unexpected or unusual sounds into an ongoing situation.
- Matching sounds to objects, or pictures.
- Locating sounds from different areas of the room.
- Responding to the 'Go game' (waiting for a sound stimulus before carrying out an activity).

The clinician should note the child's response in terms of interest, reaction time, errors, distracter behaviours and willingness to comply.

Evaluation of observational assessment and keeping records of the child's responses to specific activities is not often carried out on a formal basis, but it may be important to do so for a number of reasons:

- To chart an individual child's progress in this skill, especially when a course of listening skill therapy is being carried out.
- To compare development in this ability with changes in other areas of auditory skills development.
- To compare changes in auditory attention with speech–language production development.

A straightforward table is all that is necessary, and it can be adapted for use over various periods of time depending on the therapy management (Table 2.1).

Table 2.1 Example of an auditory skills assessment table

Name		Date of birth		Date of test or course
Auditory attention skills assessment				
Date	Time	Activity	Response	Comment
14.7.92	5 min	Go game	Distracted	Had to be restrained!
14.7.92	10 min	Sound Lotto	Many errors	Distracter behaviour

Little work has been done on providing normal developmental guidelines of auditory attentional abilities for young children probably because there are so many variables, as indicated above, related to the skill. A clinician needs to use her knowledge of how children with no speech or language deficiency respond to the various games and activities suggested above. Carrying out the assessment tasks as a group activity within a peer group setting, such as a nursery school, may help to provide comparative norms. Varying the amount and type of background noise during activities adds another dimension to the process, and may be an important factor for any one individual (see Appendix I).

Auditory discrimination

This was defined earlier as the ability to perceive small differences in the properties and qualities of sounds that fall within the same type. However, for speech and language learning purposes, this skill is applied to phonological perception and the ability to differentiate between speech sounds as the minimal units that signal meaning differences. Barton (1978; 1980) points out that this level of speech perception is distinct from acoustic perception, although the two are interrelated in that acoustic cues are necessary for the recognition of phonological features. According to Barton (1978) there is no clear-cut one-to-one relationship, although Blumstein (1980) states there is a fairly direct relationship between acoustic and phonetic perception, depending on acoustic invariance. What is of more concern to clinicians, however, is the use to which the acoustic properties are put in the classification of phonemes for language learning.

The auditory discrimination of speech sounds is an area that has undergone much empirical discussion, possibly because it lends itself to specific task performance measurement. There have been a number of reviews of the many tests and experiments relating to auditory discrimination (Barton, 1978; Monnin, 1984; Winitz, 1984) and, of these, Locke (1980) provides a clinical evaluation, looks at new ways of assessing this skill, and asks pertinent questions about what such assessments tell the speech clinician.

There are two basic procedures which have been used traditionally to measure auditory discrimination:

1. Use of a same–different paradigm where the listener has to make a comparative judgement between pairs of syllables which are either identical or which have one segment feature difference between them. Tests of this kind include the *Auditory Discrimination Test* (Wepman, 1973) and the *Templin Speech–Sound Discrimination Test* for 6–8-year-old children (Templin, 1957).
2. Use of an identification task where the listener has to identify objects or pictures whose names are phonetically similar. Tests which use this paradigm include: the *Templin Speech–Sound Discrimination Test* for 3–5-year-old children (Templin, 1957); the *Boston University Speech–Sound Discrimination Test* (Pronovost, 1974); the *Goldman-Fristoe-Woodcock Test of Auditory Discrimination*, (Goldman, Fristoe and Woodcock, 1970); the *Auditory Discrimination and Attention Test* (ADAT) (Morgan Barry, 1988).

All tests have their limitations; of those cited above all except the ADAT have been standardised on American children; several use only one-pair presentation of the stimuli and may contain phoneme pairs that are seldom confused in real speech discrimination.

A further important factor when considering the range of tests available is that those using different paradigms do not measure the same skill (Bountress and Laderberg, 1981; Cracknell, 1987). This is probably due to the fact that there are a number of processes involved in the ability to discriminate speech sounds. The 'same–different' judgement tasks involve auditory memory; the picture recognition tasks involve the ability to recognise the picture and to match it with the given word, thereby assuming some degree of linguistic knowledge. The judgemental tests are difficult to use with young children who may not have the concept of 'same' versus 'different', and the word vocabulary of the picture tests frequently contain words which are unfamiliar to the children. Barton (1978) and Owens (1961) found that wordlists of familiar words were more intelligible and therefore less likely to be confused in tests of this kind. In an evaluative study of the ADAT, Strickland (1992) found that children in language units who had poor vocabularies made more errors on the word-pairs where one or both of the words had to be taught. Their overall error score on the tests could not therefore be entirely ascribed to poor discriminatory ability.

Both Locke (1980) and Monnin (1984) advocate the need to assess auditory discrimination using the articulatory errors produced by the child, and Locke (1980) and Winitz (1984) suggest various assessment and diagnostic therapy procedures for achieving this. However, the clinician has to make a number of decisions for any individual child: whether to make inferential judgements on the child's discriminatory ability from subjective procedures; to select one or more of the standardised tests (such as those cited above) and base therapy decisions on those, or to combine both.

Subjective procedures may involve a number of activities and may follow on from those used to assess attention, but they should be based on sound theoretical principles. It is important that the clinician aims to compare the child's perceptions of his own internal articulatory form (the output lexicon) with the adult's surface form (the internal lexicon (see Hewlett's (1990) model, described above). The child may 'hear' phonetic distinctions in adult speech, but may not perceive them to be phonologically salient. For example:

> During a period of hypothesising, the child consistently is saying [w] in place of /r/; he is customarily treating them as equivalent. Why then should the child not ignore their differences in the adult's speech as he does in his own? (Locke, 1980, p. 456).

A clinician wishing to check whether the child can perceive this, or any other distinction can use what Locke (1980) calls the ABX design: using two glove puppets, the clinician explains that the puppets can talk then makes one puppet 'say' one sound and the other a contrasting sound. The child is then asked, 'Which one said i.e.....?'.

The sounds used can be single phonemes or simple syllables containing the desired contrast, either initially or finally, but it is helpful if the clinician uses a number of different pairs of sounds (including those the child *does* have contrastively) to check other variables, such as understanding of the task, motivation, attention and memory.

This type of assessment has been carried out with children aged from 3 years and with varying types and degrees of speech and language disorder. Variations of presentation include using sound pictures (Pope and Lancaster, 1990) to represent single phonemes; 'monsters' with nonsense-syllable names; and letter shapes linked with the required phoneme. (All these can later be used for auditory therapy).

The child's responses are noted in terms of error confusions, delayed response, requests for repetition, and the interesting answer to the question *'Which puppet said ...? — 'They both did!'*.

As noted above, responses can be formalised into a table which then acts as a record of the assessment over time and change in performance where auditory skills training is carried out and re-assessed. The record table may also assist the clinician to decide whether more standardised testing is needed, and/or to compare the results from both kinds of assessment (Table 2.2).

Table 2.2 Record of auditory assessment over time

Name			
Auditory discrimination assessment			
Date of birth			
Date	*Contrast*	*Response*	*Comment*
14.7.92	/s/ versus /f/	Many error responses	Did not seem able to understand task
21.7.92	/ki/ versus /ti/	50% correct	Asked for repeats

Other implications for therapy

The clinician must evaluate her ability to interpret the child's responses in terms of auditory skills and, according to her findings, make a reasoned decision about further assessment and/or therapy. Some specific therapy techniques involve auditory skills training; for example, phonological therapy (which includes teaching metaphonological awareness

(Howell and Dean, 1991) and homophony confrontation (Grunwell 1981; 1985)) requires some auditory discrimination assessment and training with the focus of such training on those phonological contrasts the child is unable to realise in his system.

The clinician's decisions relating to the amount and type of auditory discrimination testing needed for any one child must be taken with care. From initial observation, and possibly also from the results of attention assessments, a clinician may decide to use formal tests of discrimination. These may not pick up the child's misperceptions, especially if he has relatively mild articulation problems, and/or has discriminatory problems with only those sounds that are in error; it would therefore be important to check the error sounds in the manner suggested above. Alternatively, a clinician may decide to check only those sounds in a child's system which are erroneous in some way and miss the fact that he has problems of a more general nature.

Interpretation of standardised tests also needs careful evaluation from the clinician, using her awareness and observation of the child. For example, a standard score of –2.4 on the ADAT indicates a potential problem—of *either* discrimination *or* attention. The pilot study for the test found that it was difficult to ascertain whether errors made were due to a failure to discriminate or to a loss of attention (Morgan, 1984). Clinical trials have found that children with suspected diminished ability to discriminate between speech sounds are also reluctant to concentrate on the test, and use a variety of distracter behaviours to indicate this (Strickland, 1992). Other perceptual assessments of general and listening attention and discriminatory ability (as outlined above) have confirmed this relationship.

However, it has also been found that some children with good general attention skills perform poorly on the ADAT and it may be assumed that, for these children, discrimination ability is generally poor. The organisation of the test pairs may be used to give additional information as to which feature differences cause greatest discrimination difficulty, or which specific word-pairs, or whether word-initial or word-final differences are more or less easily perceived. Any one or more of these aspects can then be subjectively assessed further.

Auditory memory

According to Wepman and Morency (1973) auditory memory has been studied in children since 1887, by use of a variety of stimulus materials, such as digits, words and nonsense syllables. All studies have confirmed the developmental nature of this auditory skill, especially for children in the 5–8-year-old age range. As has been noted above, memory for the sequential ordering of phonemes, syllables and words relates to other aspects of overall perceptual ability. It is also linked to other aspects of memory, and one problem (among many) for the speech and language clinician is how to separate *auditory* memory from other auditory skills, and auditory *memory* from other memory skills.

There is also the question of the rationale behind testing auditory memory; how does it apply to speech and language learning? What effect does a deficiency in this skill have on the child's ability to perceive, understand, communicate? Zubrick (1984) makes the following point:

> ... the relationship between the increases in short term memory and lan-
> guage comprehension is tenuous at best ... imitation tasks will reveal what a
> listener retains and recalls, but not what is understood to be the underlying
> meaning of the sentences or words (p. 17).

She goes on to point out that children who have language and learning difficulties have frequently been found to have short-term memory deficits in the number of units they can retain. It may be important therefore for a speech and language clinician not only to test a child's limits and capabilities in this area but also to link these with levels of verbal comprehension, limits of visual and gestural memory skills and willingness to use his capacities for communicative purposes.

A reasonably well known test in this area is the *Auditory Memory Span Test*, which is 'a test of a subject's ability to recall single spoken words in progressively increasing series' (Wepman and Morency, 1973). It is standardised on American schoolchildren aged between 5–8 years and therefore needs to be interpreted with care when used with British children.

Subjective assessments can be carried out by clinicians using a variety of materials to accompany the spoken word. Setting out an array of objects or pictures of familiar but unrelated things (e.g. pencil, ball, sock, cup, comb, book, key ...) and asking the child, *'Give me the ... and the ...'* is a well known and used strategy.

The number of objects can gradually be increased, as can linguistic variations, *'Give me the red book, the big key and the long pencil'*. (This type of task progresses naturally to verbal comprehension tests, either formal standardised — the *Reynell Language Developmental Scales* (Reynell, 1986), for example — or informal assessments of the clinician's own devising). It is important to know how many objects the child can be expected to remember at what age; as Wepman and Morency (1973) point out, this ability is age-related. As mentioned earlier, carrying out this activity in game form in a peer group setting with normal hearing/speaking children could provide some subjective indications of how the speech–language-impaired child performs in comparisons with his peers.

Other assessments of auditory memory include:

• Asking the child to repeat digits, or to find the required numbers from a set of plastic numbers.

- Hide-and-seek-type games where the child is instructed to find a number of hidden objects or pictures (this game usually takes some time and tests the child's memory over longer timespans than the few seconds needed for immediate recall).
- Carrying out sequential instructions.

A formalised table of the child's performance can be devised as for attention and discrimination tasks (Table 2.3).

Table 2.3 Formalised record of a child's performance in assessment of auditory memory

Name	Date of birth		
Auditory memory assessment			
Date	Type of task	Response	Comment
14.7.92	Objects in array	Up to 3 correct consistently	Not always in correct order
21.7.92	Hide-and-seek	Many errors	Distracted

In planning and organising assessments, the clinician relies primarily on her initial observations of the child, preferably in a number of different environmental situations, such as the clinic, the home, or the nursery. From these first perceptual judgements of the child's behaviour, the type and amount of assessment of auditory skills can be planned and carried out. The focus of these tests will vary, as will their interpretation and the subsequent therapy based on the findings. Some children will need only a little directing of their auditory attention for the other skills to be realised spontaneously; others will need much training in all skill areas. The clinician must use her own eyes and ears in all her interactions in order to continually monitor the child's progress and to cater for his needs.

Case study: Tommy

Tommy presented with a severe phonological disorder consisting of a much-reduced sound system. Assessment of his auditory attention, discrimination and memory was carried out, using a variety of means.

Attention

In pre-school years Tommy was described as 'hyperactive' with very poor concentration and limited ability to attend to tasks even of his own choosing for more than a few minutes. At age 5;0 he was classified as being between Reynell stages 1 and 2 (Cooper, Moodley and Reynell, 1978). Assessments carried out between ages 3–5 years gave the following profile:

- 'Go-game' — difficult to condition; little attention paid to verbal command.
- Sound-to-picture matching — poor, distracter behaviour noted.
- Sound location games (in group) — little response, tended to distract neighbours.
- Musical instruments matching — unable to match sounds.

Tommy was given a number of hearing tests, but until he was aged 5 years was found to be difficult to test and the results were considered inconclusive. There was no significant history of upper respiratory tract infection. He was a very active lively child, described by his parents as 'jittery' and his nursery worker as 'meddlesome'. Therapy concentrated on improving general attentional and listening skills.

Discrimination

Assessments of this skill were not attempted until Tommy was aged 6;9, and he was one of the children used in the pilot study for the *Auditory Discrimination and Attention Test* (Morgan, 1984). His score on the experimental version of ADAT was –3.4, and it was noted that his areas of failure in discrimination concerned the fricative and affricate group. He had few errors on the /t/ and /k/ distinction, which was considered unusual, as his phonological system at that time consisted of velar substitutions for all alveolar sounds, both stops and fricatives. Further subjective testing using pairs of finger puppets and nonsense syllables gave the following results:

- /ta:/ versus /ka:/ — 100% correct discrimination
- /ka:/ versus /sa:/ — approximately 70% correct
- /ta:/ versus /sa:/ — approximately 50% correct
- /sa:/ versus /fa:/ — very few correct
- /sa:/ versus /a:/ — very few correct
- /fa:/ versus /a:/ — none correct.

It would seem therefore that although Tommy substituted velar stops [k] and [g] for all the following: /t,d,s,z,f,v, , ,/ he *was* able to discriminate between velar and alveolar stops, but unable to realise them contrastively (indicating a motor production problem); but he was *not* able to discriminate between the fricatives (indicating a perceptual problem for this group as a whole). The stop versus fricative distinction seemed to be emerging perceptually at this time of testing.

Therapy focused on the discrimination of the fricatives as a result of these assessments and, after 3 months, Tommy was re-assessed. His results showed considerable improvement in discriminatory ability, but there was little concomitant improvement in his speech production; he still used velar substitutions, although some of these were now inconsistent velar fricatives! The implications for Tommy's speech–language diagnosis are beyond the scope of this chapter to discuss, but see Morgan Barry (1989) and Stackhouse and Wells (1992).

Auditory (memory)

The *Auditory Memory Span Test* was administered when Tommy was aged 7;5, but he was unwilling to complete it. Informal assessment of his memory span using the activities outlined above showed him to be able to be consistently accurate for four items only. His visual sequencing skills, as tested on the *Illinois Test of Psycholinguistic Abilities* were found to be within normal limits.

Other tests carried out between ages 4–7 years were *Reynell Language Development Scales*, *British Picture Vocabulary Scales*, and the *Weschler Intelligence Scale for Children*.

On each of these Tommy was found to be functioning at approximately one or two standard deviations below the norm, but the general impression given by the professionals who interacted with him during this time was that he was performing below the level of his ability.

Appendix

An Auditory Skills Battery

This is a perceptual assessment which aims to cover a number of perceptual cognitive skills related to auditory attention, discrimination and memory. Because it assesses a multi-process construct it is difficult to measure objectively and therefore to standardise and to achieve a reasonably high level of inter-tester reliability. However, it can be used effectively by a clinician who is aware of her own expectations of children's performance in activities of this kind, and who has a good appreciation of how normal speaking children of various ages would perform. The assessment allows for differential 'scoring' according to the child's type of response; the distinctions being made between the different aspects of auditory perceptual skill should be assessed separately by the clinician. Allowance is also made for verbal comprehension in the scoring.

There are four simple tasks which can be carried out over a number of sessions. These are:

1. Toy play.
2. Toy play with other distracters.
3. Toy play with cassette music as background.
4. Toy play with verbal background.

Task 1

Aims

To focus attention from visual distractions.
To assess discrimination at simple word level.
To note response to verbal requests, involving memory and comprehension.

Equipment

A large jar containing a small (quiet) bell, 3 bricks, a dog, a small doll, a car.

Method

Tip toys out of the jar, and play with them with the child, naming them if necessary. Allow child to play for a few minutes then remove bell. At suitable intervals carry out the following:

- Call child's name.
- Ring bell behind back.
- Ask: *'Where's the car?' 'Where's the doll?'*.
- Request: *'Put one brick in the jar' 'Put the doll on the brick' 'Put the dog and the bell on the bricks'*. All activities may be repeated once.

Observation and scoring

Note the child's reaction time to the auditory input, involvement with the toys (and level of symbolic play), appropriate or inappropriate response to verbal input.

Score: No response = 0; Inappropriate = 1; Appropriate but slow, or following repeat = 2; Appropriate = 3. Circle any words which carried an erroneous response. Note the relationship of these words to the child's phonological system. Note any verbal response of the child. Maximum potential score = 21 (7 responses).

Task 2

Aims

To focus attention from visual distractions.
To note change in auditory attention with increased linguistic complexity.
To further assess simple discrimination at word level.
To introduce a non-contextual verbal request.

Equipment

As above, plus small teddy bear, teddy-sized bed, soft ball, 2 more bricks.

Method

Allow child to play with the toys, noting reaction to new ones. At suitable intervals carry out the following:

* Ask: *'Where's the bell?' 'Where's the doll?' 'Where's the car?' 'Where's the bear?'* (amend to 'teddy' if no response to last request).
* Request: *'Put all the bricks together' 'Can the doll sit on top of the bricks?' 'Give the ball to teddy'.*
* Suggest: *'Give the dog a ride in the car' 'Teddy's sleepy'.*
* Ask: *'What can you see out of the window?'*

Observation and scoring

Note: child's attention level as linguistic complexity increases, response to verbal input as above, score as above. Maximum potential score = 30 (10 requests).

Task 3

Aims

To focus attention from both visual and auditory distractions.
To continue discrimination at word level.

Equipment

Toys as above, plus cassette and tape of non-vocal music.

Method

Play tape at moderately soft intensity level. Carry out the following requests:

- *'Put the car behind the bricks.'*
- *'Put the ball under the bed.'*
- *'Make teddy dance to the music.'*
- *'Can you clap to the music?'*
- *'Make the doll clap to the music'.*

Observation and scoring

Note the child's response to the tape when first introduced and when attention directed to it, amount of distraction the tape produces, child's motor and rhythm response, responses and scoring as before. Maximum potential score = 15 (5 requests).

Task 4

Aims

To focus attention from other speech signal distractions.
To assess specific discriminations.

Equipment

As above, but substitute a tape of speech from an adult radio programme (i.e. of low interest and inappropriate language level for the child).

Method

Play tape at moderately soft intensity level; make the following requests:

- *'Show me the ... bed/bell/bear'*
- *'Give me the ... doll/ball/dog*
- *'Where's the ... car/jar?'*
  (NB. Present these words in random order).

Observation and scoring

Note the child's reaction to the tape, the responses to *each* word of the requests. Score as above. Maximum potential score = 24 (8 word requests).

SCORE PROFILE

Name	Date of birth	Date(s) of assessments	Comments

Auditory skills assessment battery

Test 1 scores				Test 2 scores				Test 3 scores				Test 4 scores			
0	1	2	3	0	1	2	3	0	1	2	3	0	1	2	3
Totals				*Totals*				*Totals*				*Totals*			

It would be useful to total the number of types of response: number of 0 scores = number of non-responses; number of 1 scores = number of inappropriate responses; number of 2 scores = number of slow responses; number of 3 scores = number of appropriate responses. These plotted on the above table will give a profile of the child's auditory perception ability according to the assessments administered.

References

Aram, D. and Nation, J. (1982) *Child Language Disorders*. USA: CV Mosby

Aten, J., Caligiuri, M. and Holland, A. (1982) The efficacy of functional communication therapy for chronic aphasia patients. *Journal of Speech and Hearing Disorders*, 47, 93–96

Baddeley, A. (1986) *Working Memory*. Oxford: Oxford University Press

Barton, D. (1980) Phonemic perception in children. In: Yeni-Komshian, G., Cavanagh, J. and Ferguson, C. (eds). *Child Phonology, Vol. 2 Perception*. New York: Academic Press

Blumstein, S. (1980) Speech perception: an overview. In: Yeni-Komshian, G., Cavanagh, J. and Ferguson, C. (eds). *Child Phonology, Vol. 2 Perception*. New York: Academic Press

Borden, G. and Harris, (1980) *Speech Science Primer*. Baltimore: Williams & Wilkins

Bountress, N. and Laderberg, M. (1981) A comparison of two tests of speech sound discrimination. *Journal of Child Disorders* 14, 149–156

Cooke, J. and Williams, D. (1985) *Working with Children's Language*. Bicester: Winslow Press

Cracknell, S. (1987) A theoretical comparison of two tests of auditory discrimination. Unpublished BSc dissertation. UCL/NHCSS

Daniloff, R., Schuckers, G. and Feth, L. (1980) *The Physiology of Speech and Hearing*. New Jersey: Prentice Hall

Elbert, M. and Geirut, J. (1986) *Handbook of Clinical Phonology*. San Diego: College Hill Press

Goldman, R., Fristoe, M. and Woodcock, R. (1970) *The Goldman-Fristoe-Woodcock Test of Auditory Discrimination*. Circle Pines

Grunwell, P. (1981) *The Nature of Phonological Disability in Children*. New York: Academic Press

Grunwell, P. (1985) *The Phonological Assessment of Child Speech (PACS)*. Windsor: NFER-Nelson

Grunwell, P. (1988) Phonological assessment, evaluation and explanation of speech disorders in children. *Clinical Linguistics and Phonetics* 2, 221–252

Hewlett, N. (1990) Processes of development and production. In: Grunwell, P. (Ed.). *Developmental Speech Disorders*. Edinburgh: Churchill Livingstone

Howell, J. and Dean, E. (1991). *Treating Phonological Disorders in Children: Metaphon — Theory to Practice*. London: Whurr Publishers

Jenkins, J. (1980) Research in child phonology: comments, criticisms and advice. In: Yeni-Komshain, G., Cavanagh, J. and Ferguson, C. (eds). *Child Phonology, Vol. 2 Perception*. New York: Academic Press

Locke, J. (1980a) The inference of speech perception in the phonologically disordered child. Part I: A rationale; some criteria; the conventional tests. *Journal of Speech and Hearing Disorders* XLV, 431–444

Locke, J. (1980b) The inference of speech perception in the phonologically disordered child. Part II: Some clinically novel procedures; their use, some findings. *Journal of Speech and Hearing Disorders* XLV. 445–468

Monnin, L. (1984) Speech sound discrimination testing and treating: Why? Why not? In: Winitz, H. (Ed.). *Treating Articulation Disorders: For Clinicians By Clinicians*. Baltimore: University Park Press

Morgan, R. (1984) Auditory discrimination in speech impaired and normal children as related to age. *British Journal of Communication Disorders* 19, 89–96

Morgan Barry, R. (1988) *The Auditory Discrimination and Attention Test*. Windsor: NFER-Nelson

Morgan Barry, R. (1990) Phonetic and phonological aspects of neurological speech disorders. Unpublished doctoral dissertation. University of Reading

Murphy, K. (1972) Attention and listening. In: Rutter, M. (Ed.). *The Child Who Does Not Talk*. London: Heinemann

Owens, E. (1961) Intelligibility of words varying in familiarity. *Journal of Speech and Hearing Disorders* 4, 113–129

Pope, L. and Lancaster, G. (1990) *Working with Children's Phonology*. Bicester: Winslow Press

Reynell, J. (1986) *The Reynell Language Development Scales*. Windsor: NFER-Nelson

Schwartz, R. and Leonard, L. (1982) Do children pick and choose? An examination of phonological selection and avoidance of early lexical acquisition. *Journal of Child Language*, 9, 319–336

Strickland, C. (1992) A clinical evaluation of the Auditory Discrimination and Attention Test. Unpublished BSc dissertation. UCL/NHCSS

Stackhouse, J. and Wells, W. (1992) Psycholinguistic assessment of developmental speech disorders. *NCHSS Work in Progress* Volume 2

Tallal, P. and Stark, R. (1980) Speech perception of language delayed children. In: Yeni-Komshian, G., Cavanagh, J. and Ferguson, C. (eds). *Child Phonology, Vol. 2 Perception*. New York: Academic Press

Templin, M. (1957) *Certain Language Skills in Children*. Minneapolis: University of Minnesota Press

Wepman, J. (1973) *The Auditory Memory Discrimination Test (Revised)*. Chicago: Language Research Association

Wepman, J. and Morency, A. (1973) *The Auditory Memory Span Test*. Chicago: Language Research Association

Wilcox, K., Daniloff, R. and Ali, L. (1984) Speech sound discrimination in /s/-misarticulating children. In: Daniloff, R. (Ed.). *Articulation Assessment and Treatment Issues*. San Diego: College Hill Press

Winitz, H. (1984) Auditory considerations in articulation training. In: Winitz, H. (Ed.). *Treating Articulation Disorders: For Clinicians By Clinicians*. Baltimore: University Park Press

Zubrick, A. (1984) Attending, listening and comprehending. *New Zealand Speech-language Therapists Journal, 15–29.*

Chapter 3
Assessment of voice quality: the Vocal Profiles Analysis Scheme

Sheila Wirz and Janet Mackenzie Beck

Description, analysis and management of voice

The description, analysis and management of voice disorder has been an area of great interest for speech and language therapists for many years. Therapists have a great skill in perceiving and describing vocal dysfunction and in determining, both through their knowledge of voice and their knowledge of the client, the reasons for this dysfunction. It is erroneous to assume that only voice therapists have these skills. All therapists concerned with communication disorder will consider the voice quality of their clients, and most will have skills to do this well, even if these skills are poorly recognised.

In recent years there have been major advances in the development of instrumental techniques for the measurement of both physiological and acoustic aspects of voice quality. Whilst these have undoubtedly added greatly to our knowledge and have enabled more accurate and objective measurements of many aspects of vocal performance, it is unlikely that they will ever obviate the need for systematic perceptual assessment of voice quality.

There are many reasons why instrumental analysis will probably not replace perceptual assessment, not least being the high cost of instrumental techniques and the anxiety and sometimes discomfort which such techniques may cause the client. A more fundamental problem for instrumental assessment, however, stems from the very nature of voice quality. Voice quality is a more or less continuous background to speech production, dependant on an enormously complex physiological system and involving many interrelated anatomical structures. At present, it is hard to envisage any battery of physiological assessments which could fully reflect the dynamics of the whole system.

Acoustic analysis systems, too, have limitations, which make it unlikely that they will ever entirely replace perceptual assessment. An ideal acoustic analysis system would isolate parameters from the complex acoustic signal which could be directly related to physiological factors and to perceived voice quality. At present this can be attempted only for a rather restricted set of voice features. The human auditory perceptual system, on the other hand, is extraordinarily sensitive to voice quality variation and most people can be taught to make very accurate perceptual judgements which do relate to underlying physiological adjustments. Clinical practice has embraced instrumental measurement techniques with alacrity and some clinicians have begun to question the validity of their perceptual judgements. This chapter will explore the ways in which voice can be described by use of a range of tools, will reassert the value of perceptual judgements and then describe the *Vocal Profile Analysis Scheme* (VPAS).

It is not the purpose of this review to describe voice assessments for all types of voice pathology; full descriptions are available in Hirano (1981) and Bacon (1987). It is, however, necessary to introduce some ideas about the clinical assessment of voice before going on to describe the VPAS. In this chapter the following topics will be discussed: the reasons for clinical assessment of voice; the selection criteria influencing the choice of voice assessment; and a description of some acoustic-based and physiologically based assessments which have clinical currency. There then follows a description of the VPAS, its reliability and applications.

Voice assessments tend to fall into three main categories.

1. Those assessments which have a physiological base, e.g. direct laryngoscopy where the ENT consultant examines the larynx and observes vocal fold action.
2. Those assessments which are acoustically based, e.g. the use of instrumentation to measure the acoustic consequences of phonatory performance and/or articulatory supralaryngeal performance.
3. Perceptual assessments which exploit the perceptual skills of listeners who have a clinical knowledge of voice pathology.

The professionals who undertake clinical voice assessments are primarily ENT surgeons and speech pathologists. Both want to describe voices so that they will be able to plan appropriate remedial strategies. They are less interested in simple descriptive assessment than in assessment which prescribes the appropriate remedial action to meet the need of an individual speaker. For example, an ENT surgeon needs to examine not only the physical state of the larynx but also take account of how the state of that larynx affects phonation. A speech and language therapist seeks not only acoustic measurements of the vocal output of clients as a yardstick against which to measure the efficacy of treatment, but she also needs to find a relationship between these acoustic measurements and the underlying physiological performance. Professional differences exist between the English-speaking world, where speech and language therapists (with their highly trained perceptual skills) work with ENT consultants and inform their medical colleagues about clients' voices, and, for example, Germany where phoniatrists, (medical physicians with an interest in voice) tend to have these highly developed skills themselves as part of their post-graduate training.

When selecting an appropriate method of voice assessment the clinician has to decide:

- What type of vocal sample should be observed, in order to most effectively highlight the aberrant voice features?
- Which components of a speaker's vocal apparatus should be examined in order that vocal performance can be assessed?
- Are instrumental procedures appropriate in assessment?

What type of vocal sample should be observed?

The clinician must ask whether an assessment of the vocal apparatus in a static position is adequate or whether a dynamic assessment is required and, if the latter, what length of vocal sample is required? Would steady state vowels give sufficient information or is a longer sample of speech needed to provide a long enough vocal sample?

The type of vocal sample to be assessed will vary from steady breathing with no vocalisation, through steady state vowels, to continuous spoken samples. The clinician must decide which vocal sample would be most appropriate for the assessment requirements of the specific client. The selection of an assessment procedure will reflect this decision.

Which components of a speaker's vocal apparatus should be examined?

Just as different length of vocal samples are chosen for the assessment of different laryngeal pathologies so, too, the level of the vocal tract to be assessed varies, depending on the needs of the assessment. Thus, for some pathologies, assessment of laryngeal performance will be required, e.g. in examining polyps/nodules. In others, supralaryngeal examination is required, e.g. looking at resonance disturbances of hearing-impaired speakers. In yet others it will be important for the clinician to examine both laryngeal and supralaryngeal performance of the speaker under scrutiny. Some routine physiological assessments, e.g. fibre-optic examination of the larynx, in the hands of a skilled user, give full and useful information about the state of the vocal folds, but very limited information about the supralaryngeal area. The vocal output of a client under fibre-optic examination is not typical of his usual vocal performance.

Are instrumental procedures appropriate?

Assessments which are predominantly physiological in nature aim to explain phonatory performance by assessing the physiological (and anatomical) adjustments of the vocal tract; for example, the interaction between larynx and pharyngeal state or between nasopharyngeal sphincter action and tongue root position and other similar relationships.

Such physiologically based techniques have aided our understanding of the phonatory mechanism considerably. Other physiological assessment procedures which are sometimes used involve electromyography where muscle activity is monitored and measured. Again, whereas such techniques may provide useful research data, they have little clinical currency. There are also various procedures in current use which examine the acoustic characteristics of voice. Some concentrate on waveform analysis and can be considered analogous to those physiological procedures which assess laryngeal function only. Others are concerned with the total voice signal of a speaker's output and can be considered analogous to those physiological procedures which examine both laryngeal and superlaryngeal features.

Procedures which analyse the voice signal fall broadly into three groups:

1. Those which examine parameters related to fundamental frequency.
2. Those which examine parameters related to vocal intensity.
3. Those which examine spectral features.

The emphasis of this volume is to reassert the importance of perceptual assessment and to address the understandable concern that perceptual assessments of voice lack the rigour of instrumental assessments.

Rigour is provided by the theoretical basis of the assessment and the skill of the assessor in selecting and executing the procedure. Unskilled users of both instrumental and perceptual tools will achieve poor assessments, whereas skilled users can achieve good assessments. In this volume the term 'perceptual assessment' is used rather than 'subjective assessment'. The thesis of this chapter is that trained users of a carefully theoretically grounded perceptual assessment scheme can achieve a high level of replicability and that replicability is a basic consideration in determining whether a clinical assessment tool is reliable. Perceptual skills which have become honed by training and practice can become highly replicable and in these terms highly reliable.

Perceptual assessment

There exists a wide range of perceptual assessment techniques, some published and others 'in-house'. The four principal published perceptual assessments of voice in wide clinical use include:

- The *Buffalo Profile of Voice Disorder* (Wilson 1987).
- The *Missouri Profile of Voice Disorder* (Wilson 1987).
- The GRBAS (Hirano 1981).
- The *Vocal Profile Analysis Scheme* (Laver et al., 1981).

Other perceptual schemes are available, for example, Hannarberg (1986) has made strenuous efforts to relate standardised rating procedures to acoustic correlates. However, this Swedish procedure has not been widely adopted in the English-speaking world. In addition many centres have in-house assessments where clinicians achieve congruence of perceptual judgements in their use of the assessment. This congruence is probably as a result of working together rather than any intrinsic feature of the assessment.

Any comparison of these four schemes must take into account criteria such as:

- The replicability of the assessment.
- The interjudge reliability.
- The ease of administration.

The Buffalo and Missouri profiles of voice disorder

The *Buffalo Profile of Voice Disorder* (Wilson, 1987) and the *Missouri Profile of Voice Disorder* (Wilson, 1987) have formalised the style of 'in-house' assessments as described above. They suffer similarly from the great disadvantage of not having tape-recorded examples of the parameters which they specify, nor close definitions of the scalar points of their scales. This means that, despite the ease with which these assessments can be administered, replicability and interjudge reliability cannot be guaranteed.

The GRBAS

Isshiki and colleagues (1966, 1969, 1970) attempted, by use of the Osgood Semantic Differential Technique, to explore the psychoacoustic phenomenon of hoarseness. They selected 17 polar opposite pairs of adjectives, made a tape of 16 'hoarse' voices and asked experienced listeners to rate the voices, using the prescribed adjectives. He found that four factors emerged as significant in the rating of hoarseness:

R = rough
B = breathiness
A = asthenic
D = degree

He suggested rating pathological voices by use of a four-point scale (0 = normal; 1 = slight presence; 2 = moderate presence; 3 = extreme presence) for these four factors. Thus, R3 A0 D1 (means extremely rough, not asthenic).

The work of Isshiki was further developed by the Committee for Phonatory Function Tests of the Japan Society of Logopedics and Phoniatrics as the GRBAS scale for describing voice abnormality; thus:

G (grade) 'degree of abnormality'
R (rough) 'irregularity of fold vibration'
B (breathy) 'air leakage in the glottis'
A (aesthenic) 'lack of power'
S (strained) 'hyper functional state' (Hirano, 1981, p 83).

The Japan Society of Logopedics suggests that these five factors can each be rated on a four-point scale 0–3 and give a tape-recorded example of the five factors with different scales of severity. This ensures that the GRBAS scale, unlike the Buffalo or Missouri, has some degree of reliability of use. Comments upon a speaker's voice made by use of the GRBAS are primarily comments on laryngeal function with little attention being paid to supralaryngeal parameters. Set against this disadvantage must be the fact that, once a listener has learned the GRBAS scheme, it is very quick and easy to administer.

Subtelny (1975) devised an assessment procedure specifically for hearing impaired speakers which accounted for laryngeal and supralaryngeal parameters. She specified clearly in both written form and through taped examples the terms used in her 'speech assessment', and the scalar degrees for each parameter. Her assessment includes a training tape to train the perceptual reliability of the user. The interjudge and intrajudge reliability of perceptual ratings by staff at NTID using this scheme was reported to be high (Subtelny 1975; Whitehead, 1976).

One of the difficulties of reviewing the existing assessment procedures or of evaluating descriptions used is that there is a lack of common agreement as to what constitutes voice. This chapter has used 'voice quality', 'voice characteristics' and 'vocal characteristics' synonymously. As Monsen (1979) says, 'voice quality' is a rather ill-defined term:

> For the phonetician, 'voice quality' is a technical term and refers to perceptual attributes pertaining to the way the vocal folds vibrate, for example, the laryngeal gestures. In this technical sense it is separate from qualities of speech which derive from articulation. However, while it may be true that a phonetician can listen to a word and separate the poorly executed gestures of the larynx from those of other speech articulators, most listeners probably cannot (Monsen, 1978, p. 286).

Here, Monsen is probably expressing a concern felt by many listeners and goes some way towards explaining the inefficiency of some perceptual assessment procedures. VPAS uses the term voice quality, a full definition of the term is given below.

The Vocal Profile Analysis Scheme

One of the reasons why there are these confusions of terminology in the literature is that phonetic theory has provided us with few tools with which to attempt the task of describing parameters (or groups of parameters) such as voice quality. Laver (1968, 1980, 1990) is one of the few phoneticians who have addressed this question. He says:

> In this broader approach, the view that is taken of the linguistic accountability of phonetic theory is that phonetic theory should be responsible for describing all recurrent, patterned, phonetic activity that characterizes the spoken language of the speech community concerned (Laver, 1980, p. 5).

Laver (1980), following earlier phoneticians from Sweet (1890) to Abercrombie (1967), provides the first really comprehensive phonetic description of voice quality by specifying laryngeal and supralaryngeal parameters of voice quality.

The VPAS arose primarily from Laver's early work on the phonetic description of normal voice quality (Laver 1968, 1980, 1981 – with some input from the earlier work of Wirz on deaf voice quality (Wirz, Subtelny and Whitehead, 1980)). Development of the scheme is outlined in Laver et al. (1981), reprinted in Laver (1991), and fuller descriptions can be found in Wirz (1987) and Mackenzie Beck (1988).

The VPAS was developed in an attempt to overcome some of the problems associated with previously existing schemes for voice analysis and is designed to allow the analysis of both normal and disordered voices. It is rather different from most other perceptual methods of voice analysis in three important respects.

Firstly, it moves away from the narrower traditional use of the term 'voice quality', to mean only phonatory and perhaps velopharyngeal factors. Voice quality is defined much more broadly, following Laver (1980) as 'the characteristic auditory colouring of an individual speakers voice' (p. 1). The VPAS, therefore, looks at the contribution of the whole vocal apparatus to voice quality and analyses the ways in which habitual adjustments of any part of the vocal apparatus may colour an individual's voice. This approach reflects the importance of the interrelationships between the various parts of the speech production system.

A second crucial feature of the VPAS is that all voice features are compared with a specified neutral baseline, rather than with some notional idea of normality. Given that norms for voice quality parameters vary considerably from one accent grouping to another (Esling,

1978), the use of a clearly defined, non-accent-specific neutral baseline gives the scheme a much more objective base. It also means that judges from different geographical areas will not make different judgements as a result of their different expectations about what is normal for the speech communities with which they are most familiar. The neutral baseline is a perceptual quality which is defined in terms of its acoustic and perceptual correlates. Deviations from neutral can be judged both qualitatively and quantitatively.

The third feature of the VPAS is that the overall impression of voice quality is seen as resulting from various potentially independent components, or *settings* (Honikman, 1964). These settings (see further discussion below) can be combined in different ways, which allows the differentiation of a much wider range of voices than is possible with holistic schemes, where single labels are used to describe the overall voice output. Any scheme which uses a single label for overall voice quality is limited by the difficulty most listeners experience in trying to memorise even a relatively small number of key voice qualities, and in using them to classify other voice samples. This was demonstrated most clearly in an extensive study conducted by Wynter and Martin (1981).

The remainder of this chapter aims to present:

- The main principles of the VPAS, focusing on the concept of settings.
- The procedure used when completing an analysis.
- Potential sources of voice quality.
- The reliability of the scheme.

Settings

In a speaker with a standard vocal tract anatomy, a 'setting' reflects a long-term tendency to make a particular type of muscular adjustment of the vocal apparatus. This will contribute to the characteristic voice quality of that individual. Settings, in other words, can be seen as long-term-average configurations of the vocal apparatus, around which the short-term movements necessary for the articulation of phonetic segments are made.

The neutral setting

The neutral setting in the VPAS is the baseline against which all voices are compared for the supralaryngeal vocal tract. The neutral setting is achieved when the long-term-average shape of the vocal tract is as close as possible to a tube with equal cross section along its whole length. To achieve the neutral setting the following factors must be true:

- The lips must not be protruded, spread or rounded.
- The jaw must not be protruded, unduly open or closed.
- The tongue body must lie centrally within the oral cavity, with a long-term-average posture as for [ə].
- There should be no constriction of the pharynx.
- The larynx should be neither raised nor lowered.
- Segments which are conventionally alveolar should have an alveolar place of articulation.
- Audible nasality should only be present where it is phonologically required.

A neutral phonation type, which corresponds to what Hollein (1971) has called 'modal voice' can also be defined as follows:

- Only the true vocal folds are involved in phonation.
- Vibration should be regularly periodic.
- Vibration should be efficient in air use, with full glottal adduction, without audible friction.

The acoustic correlates of the neutral setting can be clearly defined, at least for standard male vocal tracts, and Laver (1980) presents a full discussion of these correlates.

Non-neutral settings

Three broad classes of non-neutral setting may be identified. The first class, which may be called *configurational settings*, includes all long-term-average adjustments of the configuration of the vocal apparatus. There may be changes in the length of the vocal tract, as in lip protrusion or lowered larynx settings. There may be changes in the cross-section of the vocal tract at any point, as in raised/fronted tongue body settings where the tongue body is adjusted towards the hard palate. Changes in the habitual setting of the velopharyngeal system may result in more or less nasal resonance and changes in the configuration of the larynx will result in different phonation types. The second class of settings, *articulatory range settings*, concern the habitual range of lip, jaw or tongue movements used by a speaker, which may be just as characterising as the configurational settings used. Finally, it is useful to comment on the degree of generalised tension which is habitually used, hence the *overall tension settings*.

Procedures for completing a vocal profile analysis

The way in which the VPAS works may best be illustrated by summarising the steps involved in completing an individual's vocal profile. Good

quality tape-recording of a speech sample is essential, since some settings are particularly prone to distortion by common tape-recording
faults. Tape hiss, for example, may mask or mimic whisperiness or audible nasal escape. As with segmental phonetic analysis, visual cues may
be valuable in confirming auditory judgements, but are not essential
for a trained judge. Choice of speech samples (reading, spontaneous
speech, etc.) will obviously vary according to the aims of the analysis,
but in all cases the sample should be of reasonable length. It is not possible to abstract long-term-average articulatory tendencies from a sample of much less than 40 seconds, although some features, such as
phonation type, may be analysed from shorter samples.

The VPA protocol form

The development of the protocol form, shown in Figure 3.1, was seen
as a crucial factor in making the scheme maximally efficient in both
clinical and research contexts. The form is designed to reflect the
underlying phonetic theory in as much detail as possible, without
being so unwieldy as to be unusable. The form is divided into three
main sections, allowing comment on vocal quality features, prosodic
features and temporal organisation. The vocal quality section has the
firmest theoretical base and will be used to illustrate the way in which
the protocol form is used. The vocal quality section is further subdivided into two parts: a supralaryngeal (or vocal tract) section, which is
concerned with the state of the vocal tract above the larynx, and a
laryngeal section which is concerned with the configuration, position
and performance of the phonatory system. This division is somewhat
artificial as there is clearly a degree of interdependence between the
muscles controlling the larynx and those controlling the rest of the
vocal apparatus. In spite of this, it does seem to be true that many
pathological speakers show deviations from normal which cluster predominantly in one section or another. The graphical separation, on the
form, of laryngeal from supralaryngeal settings does allow an instant
evaluation of the extent to which a client presents with either a laryngeal or supralaryngeal disorder.

The basic layout of the form encourages a two-stage process of evaluation: an initial identification of neutral versus non-neutral settings,
followed by a clarification of the direction and degree of any deviation
from the neutral setting. On the left-hand side of the form are listed the
major categories within which deviations from neutral may occur (labi-
al, mandibular, etc). To the right of those labels the form is divided vertically into two sections, headed *First Pass* and *Second Pass*. The *First
Pass* section can be completed at an early stage in listening to the material, and allows a fairly crude judgement as to whether a voice is neutral or non-neutral for a given category. Under *Second Pass* the specific

settings within each category are listed, and the form allows the judge to specify the nature and degree of any deviation from neutral. Figure 3.1 shows the VPA Protocol form.

For most settings there are six scalar degrees of variation from neutral, ranging from the minimum which is perceptible to the maximum which is achievable with a normal vocal apparatus. The phonetic characteristics which determine the choice of scalar degree are specified quite exactly for each setting, but it may be helpful to give general guidelines for the interpretation of scalar degrees:

- Scalar degree 1: The presence of a setting is just audible.
- Scalar degree 2: The judge is confident about the presence of a setting but only at a moderate degree.
- Scalar degree 3: The strongest degree of a setting that could be reasonably expected to act as a sociolinguistic marker (exceptions to this rule are discussed below).
- Scalar degree 4: There is no doubt at all about the presence of the setting and it exceeds the normal limits of sociolinguistic markers.
- Scalar degree 5: Approaching the maximum deviation possible for a speaker with a normal vocal apparatus.
- Scalar degree 6: Reserved for the auditory effect associated with the most extreme adjustment of which the normal non-pathological vocal apparatus is capable.

This definition of scalar degree 6 is a necessary consequence of wishing to keep the scheme within the realm of general phonetic theory. It is obviously possible that a speaker with an abnormal vocal apparatus might be able to exceed this maximum, and scalar degree 6 can therefore be seen to operate as an open-ended category, including any level of a setting which exceeds the potential output of a normal vocal apparatus. In practice this seldom happens. The gloss given above for the differences between scalar degrees 3 and 4 must be treated with some caution. The real point is that this represents an auditory midpoint in the scale. Although it is true for most settings that this midpoint corresponds to the typical range of values used as sociolinguistic markers, there are one or two settings where this guideline fails. In the velopharyngeal category, for example, many accents of North American English are typified by scalar degree 4 of nasality. This serves to underline the earlier warning that neutral should not be confused with any notion of normality.

Sources of voice quality

Any speaker's habitual voice quality may arise from either of two possible sources: phonetic or organic. This scheme has its roots in general phonetic theory and is therefore based on the potential output of the

Speaker: ______ Sex: ______ Age: ______ Date of Analysis: ______ Tape: ______ Judge: ______

I VOCAL QUALITY FEATURES

CATEGORY	FIRST PASS Neutral	FIRST PASS Non-neutral	SECOND PASS SETTING	Scalar Degrees 1	2	3	4	5	6
Vocal Tract									
1. Labial			Lip Rounding/Protrusion						
			Lip Spreading						
			Labiodentalization						
			Extensive Range						
			Minimised Range						
2. Mandibular			Close Jaw						
			Open Jaw						
			Protruded Jaw						
			Extensive Range						
			Minimised Range						
3. Lingual Tip/Blade			Advanced						
			Retracted						
4. Lingual Body			Fronted Body						
			Backed Body						
			Raized Body						
			Lowered Body						
			Extensive Range						
			Minimised Range						
5. Velopharyngeal			Nasal						
			Audible Nasal Escape						
			Denasal						
6. Pharyngeal			Constriction						
7. Larynx Position			Raised						
			Lowered						
Phonation Type									
			Harshness						
			Whisper(y)						
			Creak(y)						
			Falsetto						
			Modal Voice						
Tension									
8. Supralaryngeal			Tense						
			Lax						
9. Laryngeal			Tense						
			Lax						

II PROSODIC FEATURES

CATEGORY	Neutral	SETTING	MILD	MOD	EXTREME
1. Pitch		High Mean			
		Low Mean			
		Wide Range			
		Narrow Range			
		High Variability			
		Low Variabaility			
2. Loudness		High Mean			
		Low Mean			
		Wide Range			
		Narrow Range			
		High Variability			
		Low Variability			
3. Tremor		Present			

III COMMENTS

CATEGORY	FIRST PASS Appropriate	FIRST PASS Inappropriate	SECOND PASS Scalar Degrees Innapropriate 1	2	3
1. Breath Support					
2. Continuity		Interrupted			
3. Rate		Fast			
		Slow			
4. Rhythmicality					

5. Other (including posture, diplophonia, etc.)

Figure 3.1 The VPA Protocol form

normal vocal apparatus. All settings described within the scheme may be produced by anyone with a normal vocal apparatus, by making phonetic adjustments which are under potentially voluntary muscular control. An individual may be characterised by those possible phonetic adjustments he habitually uses throughout speech.

It is clear, however, that an individual's characteristic voice quality may also be directly related to his vocal anatomy. Organic factors, such as unusual dental occlusion, vocal fold abnormality or atypical palatal volume, may all affect voice quality. At an auditory perceptual level, however, organically based voice quality settings and phonetically based settings may be equivalent, and the VPAS can be used to describe either.

Two examples may be used to clarify this point. The first involves mandibular settings. It is possible for anyone with a normal vocal apparatus to adopt a protruded jaw posture throughout speech and the auditory quality associated with such a habitual posture would be described as a protruded jaw setting. This is a setting which is often used in the stereotypic portrayal of determination. An individual with abnormal skeletal anatomy, resulting in an abnormally protruberant mandible, might produce an equivalent auditory voice quality as a direct result of his organic makeup, without making any voluntary adjustment.

A second example involves the phonation type, harsh voice, which is associated with significant irregularity of vocal fold vibration. A speaker with a normal larynx can produce extremely harsh voice by increasing laryngeal tension and adducting the vocal folds with the true folds, so as to create a very inefficient vibratory mass. Harsh voice may, in another speaker, be the inevitable consequence of a laryngeal abnormality, such as a carcinoma, where there is gross asymmetry of the mass of the two folds so that irregular vibration results even in the absence of excessive tension.

In both these examples the same auditory effect, which can be given the same perceptual label, has two alternative bases. It is clear therefore that the interpretation of any given profile must involve a knowledge of that individual's anatomical and physiological state.

How is reliability defined?

Reliability on the VPAS is defined as the ability to identify specific neutral or non-neutral settings and to rate the scalar degree to within one scalar degree of the 'right answer'.

For example in the four ratings of harshness given below, in Table 3.1, the 'right answer' is Harsh 2; attempts (a) and (b) have identified the non-neutral parameter and are within one scalar degree of the 'right answer' and are thus judged to be correct. On the other hand (c) has identified the non-neutral setting but has not scaled appropriately and is deemed to be incorrect.

Table 3.2 An illustration of two 'correct' ratings of harshness and one 'incorrect' rating

Harshness	N	1	2	3	4	5	6
'right answer'			X				
attempt (a)			X				
attempt (b)				X			
attempt (c)	X						

The 'right answer' in this context derives from a composite of agreed protocols by Laver et al. (1981), the originators of the scheme. These three listeners evaluated recordings of different speakers and carefully discussed these ratings and resolved the differences. These agreed judgements have been designated the 'right answer'. Laver et al. (1981) had high levels of agreement of 85% between different pairings.

A course participant who correctly identified and rated settings to within one scalar degree on each of the five voices on the evaluation tape (involving a total of 100 parameters) would have achieved an evaluation score of 100%. In reality, most course participants achieve between 65–75% accuracy on the evaluation tape after about 12 hours of instruction.

A perceptual analysis scheme is only of value if it can be learned. The VPAS has proven worth as a structured procedure whereby trained listeners can rate a speaker's vocal characteristics with a perceptual skill which is replicable and has both interjudge and intrajudge reliability.

A training course has been designed and to-date over 50 of these courses have been conducted by trained tutors. The training course which is usually of three days' duration includes approximately 12 hours of perceptual training. After this training most clinicians achieve around 65% accuracy on the evaluation tape described above.

When they finish their training course listeners invariably lack confidence in their perceptual accuracy and frequently feel that they are the exceptional trainee who has not achieved the expected level of perceptual skill. This is seldom the case.

The post-training evaluations of 242 course participants were examined after 13 courses held in the Australia, Canada, Ireland, Norway, the UK, and the USA. The Norwegian group was included to see if there were any obvious differences between the perceptual performance of non-native English speakers and speakers from the English-speaking world. Five tutors were involved in the teaching of these 13 courses in different pairings. It should be noted that all courses were conducted in different pairings. It should also be noted that all courses were conducted in English. Of these 242 course participants only two scored less than 50% on the post-training evaluation tape; the majority scored between 52–65% accuracy. Of these 242 evaluations there were no differences between the therapists from different countries; all, including the Norwegians, performed similarly. It is clear from the evaluation of the performance of trained users who continue to use the VPAS that this perceptual accuracy improves. Wirz (1987), Mackenzie Beck (1988) and Pengelly (1992) have demonstrated accuracy among practised users as high as 87%. There is, of course, some variation in perceptual accuracy between analyses of voices of different client groups. Ratings of speakers with poor motor control who exhibit a range of settings over a short space of time (e.g. speakers with cerebral palsy) are likely to have proportionately lower agreements between judges.

Applications of the VPAS

The VPAS provides a clear, graphic representation of an individual's voice quality settings which is quantitative as well as qualitative. The profile approach lends itself easily to many clinical and research applications. Perhaps the most obvious use is for the evaluation and monitoring of voice quality in individual clients, evaluating therapy, planning intervention strategies and describing group characteristics.

The graphic representation of a vocal profile analysis makes it very useful as a means of monitoring changes in voice quality, allowing the clinician to see at a glance, whether or not a client shows any relevant changes in vocal output. Given the danger of the perception of change of both the clinician and the client being influenced by the degree of time and effort invested in therapy, a more objective measure of change which does not involve expensive technology is clearly of great potential use.

The VPAS may be used in a variety of ways to evaluate and compare the efficacy of different intervention strategies. It lends itself to simple statistical evaluation of change in relation to population speaker norms.

The comprehensive nature of the VPAS means that it can be helpful in identifying strands of vocal behaviour which are contributing to the communication disorder, but which might otherwise be overlooked. A typical example is of the dysphonic client. There is a risk that assessment might focus on the phonatory system thus obscuring the possible presence of maladaptive articulatory postures which might indirectly affect the phonatory process. A comprehensive vocal profile analysis should highlight the presence of unusual supralaryngeal settings, such as close jaw or abnormally fronted and raised tongue body, which may need to be addressed before successful vocal rehabilitation can be achieved. The ability to take a global view of vocal output is clearly beneficial in planning intervention and may be especially helpful when dealing with client groups with which the therapist is less experienced.

It is possible to collect vocal profile data for any group of speakers and to construct a 'group profile' showing the mean scalar values for each setting; the range and standard deviation may also be relevant. This allows the establishment of normal baselines for the voice quality of any given sociolinguistic group, as well as the average voice quality characteristics for particular types of speech disorder. Clinicians must always remember that settings which are acceptable within any given speech community when assessing the need for therapy for a client. For example, a scalar degree of 3 for harshness would be a strong indication for investigation and intervention in many areas, whereas in certain urban areas of Scotland it would be expected as a typical feature of that accent of English.

The scheme has also been shown to be of value to other professions within the broader field of communication. For example aspects of the scheme have been used to examine the expression of emotion (Bezooijen, 1984), attribution of various social and personality features in cleft palate speech (van Erp, 1990) and the role of voice quality in mother–child interaction (Marwick et al., 1984). The VPAS harnesses and further develops the considerable phonetic skills of practising clinicians and provides a structure for perceptual assessment with a clearly defined theoretical framework.

References

Abercrombie, D. (1967) *Elements of Phonetics*. Edinburgh: Edinburgh University Press

Bacon, R.J. (1987) *Clinical Measurement of Speech and Voice*. London: Taylor & Francis

van Bezooijen, R.A.M.G. (1984) Characteristics and recognizability of vocal expressions of emotion. Catholic University of Nijmegen: doctoral thesis

van Erp, A. (1990) The phonetic basis of personality ratings, with specific reference to cleft palate speech. Catholic University of Nijmegen: doctoral thesis

Esling, J.H. (1978) Voice quality in Edinburgh: a sociolinguistic and phonetic study. University of Edinburgh: Ph.D. dissertation

Hannarberg, B. (1986) Perceptual and acoustic analysis of dysphonia. Karolinska Institute (Dept of Logopedics and Phoniatrics, Huddinge Hospital): doctoral dissertation

Hirano, M. (1981) *Clinical Examination of Voice*. New York: Springer-Verlag

Hochberg, I., Levitt, H. and Osberger, M.J. (1983) *Speech of the Hearing Impaired*, Baltimore: University Park Press

Hollein, H. (1971) Three major vocal registers: a proposal. *Proceedings of the 7th International Congress of Phonetic Sciences, Montreal*, 320–331

Honikman, B. (1964) Articulatory settings. In: Abercrombie, D., Fry, D.B., MacCarthy, P.A.D., Scott, N.C. and Trim, J.L.M. (eds). *In Honour of Daniel Jones*. London: Longman

Isshiki, N. (1966) Classficiation of hoarseness. *Japanese Journal of Logopedics and Phoniatrics*, **7**, 15–21

Isshiki, N., Okamura, H., Tanabe, M. and Morimoto, M. (1969) Differential diagnosis of hoarseness. *Folia Phoniatrica*, **21**, 9–19

Isshiki, N. and Takeuchi, Y. (1970) Factor analysis of hoarseness. *Studia Phonologica*, **5**, 37–44

Laver, J. (1968) Voice quality and indexical information. *British Journal of Disorders of Communication*, **3**, 43–54

Laver, J. (1990) *The Phonetic Description of Voice Quality*. Cambridge: Cambridge University Press

Laver, J. (1991) *The Gift of Speech*. Edinburgh: Edinburgh University Press

Laver, J., Wirz, S., Mackenzie Beck, J. and Hiller, S. (1981) A perceptual protocol for the analysis of vocal profiles. Edinburgh: University of Edinburgh (Dept. of Linguistics) *Work in Progress*. (Reprinted in Laver, J. (1991) *ibid*, pp 265–280.)

Laver, J., Wirz, S., Mackenzie, J. and Hiller, S. (1982) Vocal profiles of speech disorders. Medical Research Council Project No. G7811925N: Final Report

Mackenzie Beck, J. (1988) Organic variation and voice quality. University of Edinburgh: PhD dissertation

Marwick, H., Mackenzie, J., Laver, J. and Trevarthen, C. (1984) Voice quality as an expressive system in mother-to-infant communication: a case study. Edinburgh University (Dept. of Linguistics): *Work in Progress*, **17**, 85–97

Monsen, M. (1978) Towards measuring how well hearing impaired children speak. *Journal of Speech and Hearing Research*, **21**, 197–219

Pengelly, A. (1992) Voice measurements of post tracheostomised children. London: Great Ormond Street Hospital, pre-publication personal communication

Subtelny, J. (1975) Speech assessment of the deaf adult. *Journal of Academic Rehabilitation of Audiology*, **8**, 110–118

Summerfield, Q. (1983) Audiovisual speech perception, lipreading and artificial stimulation. In: Lutman, M. and Haggard, M. (eds). *Hearing Science and Hearing Disorders*. London: Academic Press

Sweet, H. (1890) *A Primer of Phonetics* (3rd edition, 1906). Oxford: Clarendon Press

Whitehead, R. and Subtelny, J. (1976) The development and evaluation of training materials to improve speech and voice diagnosis in hearing impaired adults. Paper presented at ASHA, Houston, Texas.

Wilson, D.K. (1987) *Voice Problems of Children* (2nd edition), Baltimore: Williams & Wilkins

Wirz, S.L. (1987) Vocal characteristics of deaf speakers. University of Edinburgh: PhD dissertation.

Wirz, S.L., Subtelny, J. and Whitehead, R. (1980) A perceptual and spectrographic study of vocal tension in deaf and hearing speakers. *Folia Phoniatrica*, **33**, 23–36

Wynter, H. and Martin, S. (1981) The classification of deviant voice quality through auditory memory training. *British Journal of Disorders of Communication*, **16**, 204–211

Chapter 4
Speech intelligibility and deafness: the skills of listener and speaker

Ann Parker and Sally Irlam

The speech and language therapist who works with deaf colleagues and clients needs to acquire a range of specialist skills. Depending on the requirements of the individual concerned, the focus of attention may be on the linguistic environment and/or the deaf individual's own communication skills, in sign or spoken language. The speech and language therapist may work closely with families and with other specialists, including sign language tutors, teachers of the deaf, audiology staff and other colleagues, all of whom are concerned with facilitating communication, and any of whom may also include speech intelligibility work in their remit. (See Halden and Gaughan, 1986; Parker and Wirz, 1986; Green and Rees, 1992, for more detailed discussions of the role of the speech and language therapist in this multidisciplinary field.)

Within this wide range of communication work, and among the various communication specialists who may be involved, a highly specific set of skills is needed when it is relevant to assess and work with an individual's speech sound system, with a view to enhancing speech intelligibility. It is with this range of skills that the present chapter is concerned, although the wider context—communication and deafness—is directly relevant to the discussion, and influences both approaches to assessment and results of intervention. This book is about perceptual issues in speech and language therapy and in this chapter, three specific perceptual issues are relevant to the discussion of speech intelligibility. They are: the deaf person's own perceptual basis for speech production patterns; the perceptions of the interlocutor, which have a direct bearing on the intelligibility of the spoken message; and the perceptual skills of the speech and language therapist, teacher of the deaf, or other specialist, who may need to transcribe and analyse the speech patterns concerned.

Although these three perceptual considerations may intuitively seem relevant, and their effects are anecdotally acknowledged in the literature, there has been surprisingly little attention given to their inter-relationship or to their effects on the results of assessment. For example, it is well known in the field of deafness that some deaf speakers may be difficult for inexperienced, hearing people to understand, but that with further acquaintance the speech seems to become more intelligible. This phenomenon is often mentioned, and sometimes enters the discussion when speech intelligibility is being considered. For example, Markides (1983) discusses the difference in the intelligibility of deaf children to teachers who know them and to other listeners who do not, and warns of the danger, arising from this difference, that the class teacher may overestimate the speech abilities of a child. In other words, acquaintance with a deaf speaker leads to an increase in speech intelligibility because of familiarity. Such an impression is seen as deceptive, either because it leads to an overestimate of the speaker's intelligibility to strangers or because it is interpreted as an actual improvement over time in the speech of the individual concerned.

This type of discussion would support 'error counts' of speech, which aim to gain a more objective picture, and to dismiss the effects, in descriptions of speech, of this particular form of variability. But this very variability involves a naturally existing condition for an increase in effective intelligibility. Explanation of the phenomenon of 'tuning in' by the interlocutor may provide an important key to our understanding of speech communication for deaf children. The question may not be how to dismiss these 'deceptive' effects on intelligibility, or reduce their influence on speech assessment, but how to maximise them in order to enhance speech intelligibility.

In addition to its implications for training the interlocutor (who will find the same speaker more intelligible after some experience of the speech) instead of the speaker in certain cases, there is a need to understand the nature of the speech patterns concerned, and to relate the patterns found to the variable intelligibility of different speakers. In this context a deficit model (one which attempts to find the differences from normal) may provide the least helpful type of information if the aim is to explain the intelligibility of speech, rather than the abnormality (Parker and Rose, 1990).

Communication and pre-lingual deafness

Deaf people do not form one homogeneous group, and a number of important variables are likely to affect the type of speech production patterns which they use. Among the factors affecting the deaf individual's speech are the timing of onset of deafness, the type and extent of hearing loss, the type and appropriateness of provision of hearing aids and communication support for the individual, and the attitudes to deafness of family, acquaintances and professionals who may be involved (see Gregory and Mogford, 1981; Hochberg, Levitt and

Osberger, 1983; Bamford and Saunders, 1992). A fundamental difference for the present discussion is that which divides all people who have a significant hearing loss into two distinct groups. One group comprises people who were born with a significant hearing loss, or acquired the loss before the development of speech. The other comprises people who developed spoken language before the onset of hearing loss. Members of either group may require the help with speech intelligibility, but the background linguistic issues are fundamentally different for each group (Meadow, 1980; Lysons, 1984; Kyle, 1987; Mindel and McCay, 1987).

For the first group—prelingually deaf people—the hearing loss is present throughout the period of first-language acquisition, and is a significant factor in the whole of the child's developmental experience. The status and use of 'speech' for this pre-lingually deaf group is highly variable. For a number of prelingually deaf people, speech may form the first language and primary form of communication (acquired with various levels of ease or difficulty depending on the variable factors mentioned above). As with hearing children, the particular speech form (spoken language) used will depend on the language or languages (English, French, Urdu, etc.) to which the child has had access (Quigley and Paul, 1984).

For other prelingually deaf people, speech may be only one form of communication, reserved for use with hearing interlocutors who are limited to spoken language communication, whilst a sign language is the preferred or first language. As with spoken language, the particular sign language used will depend on the language(s) to which the child has had access (British Sign Language (BSL) in the UK mainland, American Sign Language (ASL) in the USA, and so forth—see Kyle and Woll, 1985).

Although the majority of deaf children are born to hearing parents who use speech as the primary form of communication in the home (Woll and Lawson, 1980), many children have access to both spoken and signed forms of language. This may be because the parents make a deliberate change in the communicative environment so that the child has access to sign language (see, for example, Fletcher, 1983) or because the child's special educational setting provides sign language (Bouvet, 1990) or because, in spite of an exclusively 'oral' home and school policy, the child meets other deaf children and adults who use sign language (Deuchar, 1984, Kyle and Woll, 1985). It is therefore the case that many deaf children develop in a bilingual or multilingual environment, whether by natural occurrence or by design (Gregory and Hartly, 1984; Lane, 1984a; Sainsbury, 1986). It is thus not surprising that communities including deaf and hearing people use a range of communication forms which show the parallel influences of sign language (the language of the deaf community) and speech (the language of the hearing majority).

This range of communication patterns is explicable in terms of the bilingual reality of communication for prelingually deaf people, but it is complicated by the fact that whereas deaf children may be given access to sign language 'by design', it follows that they may also be *deprived* of access to either spoken or sign language. The hearing loss itself may account for much of the denial of access to spoken language (Connor, 1971), as may poor hearing aids and lack of appropriate support for the development of spoken and written communication (Ling, 1976; Gregory and Mogford, 1981; Wood et al., 1986). Access to sign language may be limited by simple lack of exposure (in that the majority of hearing people are unable to use the language fluently, see Finkelstein, 1984) or by actual policy, as in the case of education authorities and establishments which have a declared 'oralist' policy, whereby the only acceptable form of communication for language development and educational purposes is deemed to be speech (Mulholland, 1981; NAG, 1981).

This complication (the fact that the linguistic environment of the deaf child is necessarily subject to some form of manipulation, be it in the provision of sound amplification or a fundamental change in the natural linguistic environment) has provided the basis for a controversy which has raged throughout the recent history of deaf people. The situation has been perceived by a number of observers as being an example of linguistic imperialism, in the form of subjugation of a minority language and culture (sign language and deafness) by the majority, hearing people (Woodward, 1982; Gregory and Hartly, 1984; Lane, 1984b; Wilcox, 1988; Sacks, 1991).

Since the language of the majority in this context is speech, the controversy provides a complex background to considerations of speech intelligibility. Speech (one possible form of communication, and the primary form used by hearing people) has been elevated by one group to the position of the only possible vehicle for language development, and dismissed by another as oppressive or irrelevant for the deaf community. The observable reality is that some deaf people use sign language as their preferred and only form of communication, others communicate predominantly with speech and yet others—possibly the majority—function bilingually (Schlesinger, 1978; Grosjean, 1982; Gudykunst, 1988) in that they use either sign language or speech, depending on the skills of the interlocutor(s), and also have available to them a range of 'interlanguage' skills which involve simultaneous and modified use of spoken and signed forms. This latter, 'interlanguage' form, when the spoken language concerned is English, has been described variously as 'Signs Supporting English', 'Manually Coded English' and 'Pidgin Sign-English', the first two terms being relevant only for versions with a predominance of spoken language word order. (See Schlesinger and Namir, 1978; Woll, Kyle and Deuchar, 1981;

Quigley and Paul, 1984; Kyle and Woll, 1985, Padden and Humphries, 1988; Taylor and Bishop, 1991 for more detailed examinations of these issues.)

An additional factor which is relevant to considerations of speech is the fact that although the deaf person may use spoken language, whether as a preferred form or not, there will be a shift of mode, in that the individual may be relying on visual cues for speech perception to a greater extent than hearing speakers do, or may even, if the hearing loss is sufficiently profound, be functioning entirely in a visual mode. The extent to which hearing is available for speech may be a crucial factor in the individual's own speech intelligibility, and although simultaneous visual self-monitoring is not a possibility in normal communication, visual and visible cues in speech may nevertheless be the basis for the speech sound system of the individual concerned, because of the visual nature of the input model (Schlesinger, 1978; Summerfield, 1983).

Communication and acquired deafness

If the world of prelingual deafness is dominated by controversy and linguistic disagreements, that of the group with acquired deafness has suffered from the opposite problem, namely a marked lack of debate or attention (Kyle, 1987; NDCS, 1987). Recent developments in the field of cochlear implantation have increased the published information for one section of this group, but in general it is difficult to find detailed information about speech production, because attention has mostly been focused on the primary and most obvious problem of deafened individuals—their own access to the spoken word, through amplified sound and/or speechreading (Watts, 1983). The majority of this group are already adults and have established not only at least one spoken language but also an adult level of control over their own lives before the onset of hearing loss. In addition, the language used to communicate is a spoken language, in common with the majority of hearing people, with the result that linguistic prejudice (except for any which already exists because of the particular spoken language concerned) is not the issue here. The deafened individual experiences reduced ability for auditory reception of the spoken message, but retains the previous capacity to process and produce language once it is perceived. Changing the channel of input to a visual one by use of the written form immediately establishes complete understanding, because the language has not been lost.

However, communication by use of the written form is not convenient in face-to-face situations. Deafened individuals have in common with people who are born deaf the fact that for the spoken form the mode of linguistic transmission is different. The balance between auditory and visual information has changed. In effect, the input has switched from auditory (plus or minus visual) to visual (plus or minus auditory). The auditory feedback loop which provides own-speech monitoring has also changed, and it is the loss of this information which is the primary basis of the deafened individual's speech production changes (Parker, 1983).

Speech intelligibility and deafness

Given the profound differences in the effects of deafness occurring before and after the development of speech, it is not surprising that it is customary to separate the two groups when describing the effects of deafness on communication and language. However, the effects on speech intelligibility will be described here without this separation, for a number of reasons.

Firstly, the communication worker specialising in deafness may or may not specialise in working with a particular subset of deaf people (children or adults, prelingually deaf or deafened) but, even if specialising within the field, he or she is unlikely to do so exclusively. The range of adult deaf clients seeking help to improve their intelligibility (or other communication skills) is not usually restricted to one group or the other, and therefore the therapist or teacher needs to be aware of the whole range of patterns which may need description.

Secondly, the two groups are not as discrete as the above description would imply. When all of the other variables (amount of hearing, attitude to communication, appropriateness of intervention) are taken into account, there is actually considerable overlap between the two groups. For example, some children who were deafened after acquiring spoken language may have been educated in a school for deaf children and may prefer to communicate in sign language even though they are effectively bilingual. Other deafened adults may become involved as professionals in deaf issues and acquire proficient sign language for their work, also functioning in a bilingual context. On the other hand, a child who is born profoundly deaf, given excellent support and help to develop spoken language and educated with a hearing peer group may function as an adult entirely within the hearing, spoken language community. Partially hearing adults may have had the hearing loss from birth but access to spoken language may have been effective and sufficient for integration within the majority, hearing community.

Finally, there is the possibility that a prelingually deaf child or an early-deafened child may be effectively deprived of access to both spoken and sign language and may, for a variety of reasons, reach adult life without the ability to function fully in either form of language.

For these reasons, when speech intelligibility is the issue, the specialist who wishes to assess speech may do well to make no assumptions until the language and communication patterns themselves have been assessed. The full range of possibilities, and the ability to deal with them appropriately, should be known and considered.

This means that the specialist should be directly involved with the deaf community and its issues, working closely with deaf professional colleagues across the whole range of communication and languages concerned (Llewellyn-Jones and Wirt, 1988). Unless the therapist or teacher concerned is a native sign language user, work with both spoken and sign languages, in auditory and visual modes, will necessitate (in a way comparable to other bilingual settings) the involvement of deaf co-workers, and even if the focus is on speech effectiveness (of which intelligibility is a part), this should be a choice based on the client's requirements, and so not on the limitations of the service provider. The whole range of auditory-mode and visual-mode communication is relevant in assessment of speech, both in general and in some specific ways which are discussed below, and, whether the focus of work is with children or with adults, an interdisciplinary 'interlinguistic' team provides the most effective way of covering the range.

Speech production should, then, be assessed within the context of a more general assessment of communication. There are a number of other relevant considerations which will affect the outcome of assessment.

Perceptual skills of the assessor

The first of these concerns the starting point; not 'what the assessor does first', but 'what the assessor already knows'. There is a constraining circularity in speech assessment, whereby the existing skills and knowledge of the assessor (including the influence of her own first language) may prevent awareness of the patterns which are used by speakers using different systems. This is a well-attested phenomenon in second-language learning, whereby speakers of the new language find it difficult to pronounce and perceive contrastive features which are different from those in their first language. Examples of this effect are the famous 'l/r' confusion of Japanese speakers learning English, the inappropriate omission and insertion of syllable-initial 'h' in some French speakers' use of English, and the difficulty which English speakers have with, for example, French nasal vowels, with the front, close rounded vowel [y], or with Cantonese tones. These difficulties are related to the fact that the speech sounds concerned either are not found at all or are not linguistically contrastive in the first language of the speaker, and that this constrains perception and production, at least initially, of the sound patterns of the new language (see Catford, 1988; Gimson, 1989; Kelly and Local, 1989).

The purpose of 'phonetics ear-training', undertaken by linguists and phoneticians who wish to analyse the sound patterns of any language, is to provide a range of symbols for transcription purposes which is as versatile as possible, covering the whole range of known contrasts in languages (it should be noted that this, too, is a circular argument; the contrasts have to be known before the symbols can be developed, and the phonetician therefore needs to recognise new patterns for which there is, as yet, no agreed symbol; see PRDS, 1980; Duckworth et al., 1990). The body of knowledge, skills and symbols developed by phoneticians for the purpose of analysing the systems of new (to them) languages provides a starting point for speech and language therapists, and others, who wish to transcribe and describe both normal developmental patterns in children and the speech of children and adults who may have problems with development. For this reason, a requirement in the training of the speech and language therapist is a relatively prolonged programme of ear-training, to enable a level of accuracy in the analysis of speech production patterns. The phonetic problems associated with language development and breakdown may extend the known ways in which normal, adult languages use speech sound systems. This necessitates an additional element in any effective training for speech and language therapists and teachers of the deaf, involving not only practice with sounds of known languages and dialects other than that of the trainee but also work with data from children's developmental systems and from speech therapy clients with 'abnormal' systems (Grunwell, 1990). Again, there is a circular argument; the systems must be observed accurately and analysed before decisions about normality or effectiveness can be made.

The analysis itself, of course, is not trivial, and much of the focus of recent work and debate by linguists in the field of speech pathology has been in the application of general linguistic principles, after phonetic or other transcription, to the specification of rules which would generate the speech systems concerned (see Ball, 1988). This work is highly relevant to the field of deafness, and has received surprisingly little attention within the field. Nethertheless, there is also a need to examine the phonetic level in the process of assessment.

Where the systems used by deaf speakers are concerned, there is yet one more level of circularity, which may impede accurate observation and transcription, and therefore constrain every subsequent stage in the process of analysis. Deaf speakers may (and, as described below, do) use a particular range of speech sound systems which can be explained in terms of their auditory–visual perception of the normal targets concerned, but which may be overlooked by the transcriber who has not been alerted to, and trained in perceiving, the possibility of such sound contrasts and systems. Therefore, there is a third level of phonetic/linguistic training required for professional workers who are involved in assessing the speech of deaf people, and the necessary basis for this is an existing body of knowledge about the types of patterns which tend to occur. Unfortunately, there is little in the existing literature to provide this important information. The rest of this chapter is concerned with a discussion of some of the reasons for this problem, and an account of the patterns which are actually found, in an attempt to fill the gap, and provide a practical framework for the assessment of speech production in deaf speakers.

Speech patterns of deaf adults

The patterns described are taken from a corpus of data provided by a project with deaf adults (Irlam, 1982). The study of patterns in the adult population of deaf people has several advantages. Firstly, although members of the (prelingually) Deaf Community within this group may have suffered the deleterious effects of the controversies described above, the current situation is likely to be relatively stable, and the deaf adult is in a position to choose interlocutors, language and language form. In this context, observation is likely to be least clouded by controversy and pedagogical control. The speech patterns themselves are also likely to be stable, which may not be the case for children's developing language. What is observed may genuinely be described, for most adults, as the 'end-point' of any previous intervention. In this respect, the study of speech patterns in deaf adults may throw useful, and more objective, retrospective light on the claims of advocates of particular educational/rehabilitation systems. A group of deaf adults is more likely to include adventitiously deafened individuals, and therefore cover the whole range of the effects of deafness. Finally, it is possible to obtain the informed, adult consent of the individuals concerned for their anticipation in the survey, a factor which is always comforting for the researcher but in the field of deafness has particular value, especially as the opinions of the adults concerned may give useful additional information about speech and deafness.

There are also some fairly obvious disadvantages to reporting patterns found in adults. Firstly, a 'speech' project may not attract the involvement of those individuals who have been disaffected by their experience of 'linguistic imperialism' (see above). Secondly, although the analysis of stable, adult systems may offer interesesting retrospective evidence about the linguistic experiences of the speakers concerned, it does not, of itself, provide information about the developmental stages which preceded this adult form, any more than developmental processes in children's language can be inferred simply from knowledge of adult, normal phonological systems. Developing phonological systems must be studied in their own right (Grunwell, 1987). But since the end-point of the development of a deaf speaker's phonological system may not be synonymous with normal, adult

English, the synchronic study of adult, deaf speaker's phonologies may provide an important reference point for the analysis of the speech of deaf children. Accurate observation and analysis of the individual speaker's system forms the essential basis for any programme of intervention for a deaf speaker who wishes to improve intelligibility. Whilst the description of the system necessarily involves linguistic analysis, the starting point (phonetic transcription) and the end-point (explaining, eliciting and establishing normal phonetic realisations of linguistic rules) of intelligibility work with deaf people involves considerable attention to phonetic-level information (Pye, Wilcox and Siren, 1988; Parker and Rose, 1990). The accuracy of the information concerned is therefore of great importance, and this depends on the observer's ability to transcribe the speech production and relate the patterns observed to the communication of the individual in a deaf and/or hearing communicative context.

An overriding limitation on the assesssor's perceptions may be lack of experience. If the observer is not familiar with, or even aware of, the types of pattern which may be produced by deaf speakers, important patterns of linguistic contrast and structure may be lost to the analysis because of the 'never-seen-before' phenomenon. In order to avoid this pitfall, the circularity described above needs to be interrupted by the provision of information from studies of deaf speakers.

Unfortunately, much of the existing published information on the subject provides only a limited basis for confidence about accuracy, because of a range of specific constraints which observers need to avoid. Ten of these limitations are listed in Table 4.1, and will be discussed in relationship to some characteristic patterns found in the speech of deaf adults.

Table 4.1 Ten avoidable constraints on the phonetic basis for speech assessment

1. Speech is studied only from an 'oralist' perspective.
2. 'Normal Adult System' (NAS) dominates the perceptions of the observer (whose transcription is limited to the 'phonemic repertoire' of his/her own language/accent).
3. Error analysis forms the basis of description.
4. The observer is limited to the phonetic repertoire provided by the IPA* chart.
5. The transcription is limited to representation of audible features.
6. Alternative realisations of NAS linguistic contrasts are not recognised.
7. Transcription and analysis are limited to segmental features.
8. The corpus of speech material elicited omits relevant features.
9. The analysis assumes an articulatory basis for patterns rather than relating them to the auditory–visual perceptions of the speaker.
10. Intelligibility is attributed only to the speaker; interlocutor and context are ignored.

*IPA = International Phonetic Alphabet.

Speech from an 'oralist' perspective

Many of the published studies of the speech of deaf people are presented from a stated 'oralist' viewpoint, and do not accept or acknowledge
the relevance of sign language (see, for example, Ling, 1976; Hochberg,
Levitt and Osberger, 1983; Markides, 1983; Nittrouer and Hochberg,
1985). Where deafened speakers are concerned, this would be an
unsurprising observation. This group communicate, by definition, with
speech, and there is no reason to expect a sudden change to a different
language as a result of an acquired hearing loss. In the presence of a
pre-linguistic hearing loss, however, the individual may develop language and communication forms across a range of spoken and sign language (for example, English and BSL in the UK, English and ASL in the
USA, Swedish and SSL in Sweden) and, furthermore, may use features
from the sign language concerned as an adjunct to communication in
the spoken language, as with 'Signs Supporting English' (SSE) or
'Manually Coded English' (Quigley and Paul, 1984). Any speech assessment which ignores this fact misses a number of facets of speech intelligibility for such speakers.

For example, it is often the case that a prelingually deaf adult
speaker seems not to use the voiced–voiceless contrast. Voiceless
speech sounds may be absent from the speech altogether, or the speaker may actually use no voice at all, or the contrast may be inconsistent
for a range of elicited English minimal pairs. If the 'speech' is considered as articulation patterns alone (maybe because the observer considers only this part of communication relevant, or does not know any
sign language) the assessor may conclude that the speaker is incapable
of distinguishing minimal pairs, such as 'tin/din', 'fat/vat' and
'coat/goat' in speech production, or is unaware of the phonological distinction even if the semantic contrast is known. However, in reality,
deaf speakers have a number of ways of signalling 'phonetic' contrasts
in spoken communication, by using either the equivalent lexical item
from their sign language (as in, for example, 'SSE') or finger-spelling.
Both of these forms are used by many deaf speakers to disambiguate
utterances which would otherwise be visual homophones. To the interlocutor (or speech assessor) who does not know the sign language or
finger-spelling system concerned such a speaker might rate extremely
low in intelligibility, but linguistically proficient communicators (such
as deaf people) might have no difficulty whatsoever in understanding
the speech. If this type of communication is to be assessed realistically,
the assessor needs to be in a position to perceive visual 'loan features'
from the sign language concerned. Furthermore, intervention to
improve intelligibility for some speakers (including those who are deafened, and some of the hearing interlocutors they wish to lipread) may
include the introduction of such additional visual cues to speech

perception. It may also involve discussion of alternative tactics for the deaf speaker wishing to communicate with an interlocutor who does not know the cues from sign language.

'Normal Adult System' (NAS) dominates the observer's perceptions

A second set of problems to be avoided is related to perceptual limitations of the assessor within the spoken language concerned (items 2–6 in Table 4.1). There may be a problem in assessing speech which is different from that of the assessor because of the perceptual filtering effect of the assessor's own particular linguistic system. Features which are either absent or not linguistically contrastive in the assessor's own dialect may be perceived inaccurately, or not at all. Much practical training in phonetics (an absolute necessity for this work) is designed to overcome the perceptual constraints of the transcriber's own language and accent, but there are additional considerations where deafness is concerned, which will make accurate observation of some speakers extremely difficult if the NAS of the assessor is the only frame of reference (see Pye, Wilcox and Siren, 1988, for a discussion of inter-transcriber agreement and its relevance to the speech of deaf speakers).

The most basic perceptual constraint on the assessor is the phonemic repertoire of her own dialect, if it is the sole basis for transcribing the deaf speaker. This may happen if the assessor has not received adequate practical ear-training, or if skills previously acquired have deteriorated from lack of use. The phonemic inventory of any form of normal adult English is an insufficient range for transcription of the speech of someone with a different system of contrasts. It would be comparable to transcribing, for example, French or Swahili with only the symbols for English speech sounds; even if the 'non-English' speech sounds were perceived they could not be transcribed. Where deaf speakers are concerned, this type of limitation may obfuscate the linguistic analysis, in that phonological contrasts which support speech intelligibility for the speaker concerned, provided the listener has 'tuned in' to the system, may be completely overlooked in the assessment.

'Error analysis' forms the basis of description

A related problem is commonly found in the literature on the speech of deaf people, which abounds with accounts of the 'errors' in deaf speech, and discusses 'untranscribable' features, sometimes referred to as 'distortions' because they are not found in the phonemic inventory of adult, normal English (see, for example, Levitt and Stromberg, 1983; Markides, 1983; Stoel-Gammon, 1983). Narrow phonetic transcription of the speech of deaf adults shows that many of these 'distortions' are not only recognisable speech sound contrasts in other spoken languages, but that they serve an effective contrastive function in the speech of the deaf speaker concerned (see Parker and Rose, 1990, for a further discussion of this feature of the speech of deaf people). The transcriber of this speech needs to have available the full range of symbols from the International Phonetic Alphabet (IPA) (see Gimson, 1989), including the ability to transcribe implosives, clicks and ejectives as well as egressive pulmonic airstream consonants in the whole range of possible places of articulation, and the analysis which follows needs to account for the level at which such features function in the communication of the speaker. For example, one speaker may use [b] (a voiced bilabial plosive) in contrast to [p'] (a voiceless bilabial ejective) to represent the NAS 'voice–voiceless' contrast at bilabial place, whereas another may use the differing feature (airstream mechanism) in free variation in speech, 'voice–voiceless' being either uncontrasted in any way, or contrasted in a non-speech way as described above.

Limitations of the 'IPA Chart' range

The IPA range is necessary, but not sufficient for all transcription purposes, because of the need to account for any potential speech contrast. Various writers (for example, see PRDS, 1980; Duckworth et al., 1990) provide an example of extended repertoires for the speech and language therapist, but deaf speakers produce an even wider range than this, and 'never-heard-before' phenomena cannot be prevented entirely. Symbols for commonly occurring sounds (for example, bi-dental percussive, bilabial roll, bilabio-lingual plosive) are available, and the convenience of their use may accelerate progress to the speech analysis stage, but for individual speakers phonetic transcription may require an inventive approach, with liberal use of the asterisked phonetic-descriptive footnote (see also Grunwell, 1987) or the rapid generation of a new symbol. An example is the use of a representative of NAS lateral approximant /1/, which is found in a few speakers. This is a 'voiced labio-lingual lateral roll', which involves the rapid alternation of apico-labial contact with the left and right sides of the upper lip of the speaker—possibly the result of unhelpful intervention, but in at least one observed case contrastively functional, with [1] consistently used to represent NAS /n/.

Transcriptions limited to audible features

Many studies of the speech production of deaf people have relied on an audiotape recording to produce data analysis, whether of intelligibility or 'errors' (see, for example, Brentari and Wolk, 1986, who used such a basis to compare speech intelligibility with and without manual support). However, a particularly common feature of the speech of profoundly deaf speakers is the use of the 'silent articulations' to represent phonological contrasts in the target (NAS) system. This is consistent with the mode-shift towards visual, mentioned above, which affects the speech perception and production of many speakers with a hearing loss and, if such articulatory gestures are missed by the transcriber (as will be the case if the assessor is either insufficiently skilled or relies on audiotape recording and/or acoustic measurement as the basis for transcription, when all visual information will clearly be lost), the phonological analysis may be seriously inadequate. Commonly in our data, silent articulatory gestures, clearly visible but completely inaudible, are used to represent syllable-final consonants, word-final syllables and utterance-final words, and whole utterances. Thus, their omission in transcription could lead, depending on the level of analysis used, to inaccurate representation of the syllable-final consonant system, or indeed of the word-structure or sentence-structure used by the speaker. The fact that these features are represented in a visible rather than audible form may well reduce speech intelligibility when lipreading is not available to the 'listener' (either because of the situation—as in communication by telephone or from one room to another—or because of the limited skills of the interlocutor). It does not mean, however, that the speaker is entirely unaware of them. If this were the case they would not be represented at all. It is therefore relevant for the assessor to be aware of the existence of visual representations in the speaker's 'phonology'.

Alternative realisations of NAS contrasts are not recognised

The aim of further perceptual training for the assessor, both within and outside the range of IPA symbols, is to extend the range of possible speech sound systems which can be analysed. Any particular phonetic feature which is observed may (or may not) represent an alternative phonetic realisation of a NAS contrast, which may help the speaker's intelligibility with known interlocutors, and which may explain the frequency of the 'tuning in' phenomenon, whereby barely intelligible speakers become highly intelligible after a fairly brief acquaintance. The most likely way to lose the phonetic and linguistic evidence necessary for judging a feature's phonological status is to produce a 'broad' transcription from a poor quality audiotape recording by an untrained listener, by use of an uncontrolled sample of speech which is unintelligible to the transcriber. This type of procedure (variants of which are used surprisingly often) may throw interesting light on the possible intelligibility of the speaker to naïve listeners on the telephone (the poor sound quality produced by many tape recorders providing an approximation to

the reduced band-width of the telephone) but in this era of text-tele-
phone communication this may be the least important consideration for
the deaf speaker concerned. The results of such a process are likely to
fall short of an adequate basis for phonological analysis or intervention.
Whether or not the sounds transcribed have a linguistically contrastive
function for the speaker concerned, they need to be assessed as accurately as possible because any intervention which is contemplated necessarily involves an exact understanding of the ways in which the speaker's
speech—both phonological system and phonetic realisations—differs
from normal. The appendix to this chapter provides examples of the
need for accurate transcription. (See also Pye, Wilcox and Siren (1988)
and Parker and Rose (1990) for further discussion of the ways in which
accuracy of transcription may affect the results of analysis.)

Limitation to segmental features

Another major limitation of much existing work is the omission of
appropriate material for a full non-segmental analysis. Many writers
have commented that the speech of deaf speakers differs from hearing
speakers in its non-segmental features (see, for example, Osberger and
Levitt, 1979; Horii, 1982; Stevens, Nickerson and Rollins, 1983;
Whitehead, 1983; Stathopoulos et al., 1986) but, as with segmental
analysis, the concentration has often been on phonetic 'correctness' or
normality, rather than assessing the speaker's use of linguistic contrasts.
Where features such as perceived tension level, breath control, overall
loudness and rate of utterance are concerned, a deficit-model approach
is not necessarily problematical, and the traditional categories of voice
description used by speech and language therapists are relevant, provided that the phonetic description is relatively detailed. For example,
'inadequate' breath control may involve an inadequately shallow intake
of air, or an intake which seems adequate followed by excessive outward
airflow, associated with breathy voice quality at the beginning of breath
groups and low-pitched, creaky voice (glottal fry) as the lung air reserve
is depleted, towards the end of a breath group. Alternatively, the airflow
problem may be associated with the use of airstream mechanisms which
are non-pulmonic and/or non-egressive (producing the implosives, ejectives and clicks mentioned above, which may function contrastively in
the segmental system or simply be observable as non-contrastive overall
features of speech production). It is at this, 'least linguistic' end of the
non-segmental continuum (Crystal, 1987) that observers who are
trained speech and language therapists may need least additional training, since they are familiar, through the well-established field of voice
work, with the range of phonetic variation which is possible in speech
production. Procedures are widely available for the assessment of voice
quality, and are outlined in Chapter 3 of this book.

However, the linguistic use of non-segmental contrasts (the rhythm and intonation systems of the language concerned) are unlikely to be disturbed systematically by most voice disorders in the absence of deafness. Rhythm and intonation systems are less well documented in the literature on deafness, and are less well served by existing assessment procedures. Because less attention has been paid to non-segmental aspects of speech than to segmental features, there is a less than adequate basis in the literature for either assessment or intervention. Rhythm and intonation patterns are linguistically contrastive and language-specific (see Couper-Kuhlen, 1986; Johns-Lewis, 1986). This means that a change of rhythm or of intonation may systematically signal a change of meaning, and the rules for such changes differ in different spoken languages (see Ladd, 1980). The implication of the systemic nature of these patterns is that deaf speakers, as with segmental features, may not simply produce 'errors' (and 'correct' or 'incorrect' patterns) but may be using different systems of contrast, which will enable, restrict or change contrasts of meaning at the semantic level, in comparison to the English NAS. Lack of recognition of this possibility leads to an additional difficulty, in that the speech sample elicited for analysis may not cover the range of non-segmental linguistic contrasts which need assessment. This may compound the difficulty caused by the lack of a conceptual framework for the assessor, because the data concerned may offer no challenge to the original assumption, that intonation and rhythm will be correct or incorrect.

Omission of relevant features from the speech sample

Intonation patterns provide the most striking example of the danger of omission of appropriate data from the speech sample. Intonation patterns in English are closely related to measurable changes in fundamental frequency (and are perceived by listeners as changes in the pitch of the speaker's voice). In English, for example, primary emphasis, or sentence-stress, in a phrase is usually conveyed by a change in voice pitch (fundamental frequency) within one or more syllables of the word concerned. Thus, the utterance, *'Why don't you go home?'* may be spoken in a number of different ways, emphasising any one (or more) of the constituent words in contrast with all of the others. A linguistically competent speaker of the language needs to be able to vary the pitch of the voice appropriately in order to convey the intended meaning. A speaker who is deaf may use the same linguistic rules to emphasise the primary stress, or not, and the rules may be phonetically realised in the same way, or not.

Clearly, a full description of the speaker's speech patterns must include an analysis of intonation, but an uncontrolled, spontaneous speech sample may not produce the kind of sequence which would elucidate the speaker's system. This is especially true where intonation contrasts function at discourse, rather than sentence, level, as in the following conversational sequence:

Speaker 1:   Why don't you go *home*?

Speaker 2:   I *am* going home.

Speaker 3:   *I'm* going home, too.

               Why don't *you* go home?

Speaker 4:   I'm going home *later*.

This type of sequence involves the use of 'intonational minimal pairs' (see Parker and Rose, 1990), or utterances which are identical lexically but differ in meaning because of one change in the intonation pattern. In the example above, the change involves moving the 'nucleus' of the utterance (the location of the major voice-pitch change, in this case a falling pitch, which conveys emphasis) to a different word, with a corresponding reduction in salience for the less important syllables. Intonational minimal pairs provide the simplest evidence about an individual's use of intonation contrasts, but they may or may not occur in an uncontrolled speech sample. Therefore, even if the observer attempts to analyse this aspect of the intonation system of the speaker, there may not be sufficient data for the purpose.

In order for the assessor to perceive and analyse non-segmental phonological systems a suitable discourse sample is required, and once more experience is needed (or information based on other assessors' experience) of the range of patterns (linguistic systems and phonetic realisations) which deaf speakers are likely to produce, as well as an understanding of the NAS systems concerned. Some examples of such patterns are given in Figure 4.1 (see also Parker and Rose, 1990).

Auditory–visual perception and the role of the interlocutor; types of speech

The two final points of Table 4.1 bring the discussion back to the introductory remarks of the chapter, concerning the wider context of communication and deafness, and its relationship with speech assessment. From some of the examples presented, it is apparent that 'intelligibility' may be in the eye (as well as the ear) of the beholder, and may vary considerably as a function of the beholder's experience. Deaf people may wish to communicate, when using speech, with hearing and/or other deaf people. Even the hearing group may 'tune-in' to the visible contrasts which are used, and also learn some sign language. It would therefore seem appropriate to take this dimension into account in assessment, and to incorporate an awareness of the variable range of

Perceived voice quality, pitch and timing of each syllable, transcribed by trained listeners and checked with objective measurement of voice fundamental frequency and duration, provides a basis for analysis of the role of non-segmental features in speech communication, provided that the speech sample includes the opportunity for a range of intonation contrasts. Unlike voice fundamental frequency printouts, which are generally continuous except for voiceless segments and pauses, such transcription separates each syllable to enable an impressionistic representation of relative syllable length. Each example in Tables 3A and 3B involves the sequence.

"I think they're on the chair. No... under the chair."

1. NORMAL ADULT SYSTEM (NAS)

Word stress (the basis of rhythm) is conveyed primarily by additional length for stressed syllables, with briefer, reduced or "weak" forms for the unstressed syllables. Further emphasis (sentence stress, or primary stress) is enabled by a pitch change, falling for the first occurrence of "chair" and for "under", and rising for "No".

Loudness is relatively constant, and does not form the primary basis for either type of contrastive stress.

Examples 2-4

Differences from the NAS operate mainly at phonetic level. The central linguistic systems of timing and pitch contrasts (rhythm and intonation) are maintained despite marked overall differences in voice quality, pitch range, timing or loudness, but speakers may nevertheless convey unintended attitudes because of these phonetic changes.

2. "Creaky voice" interferes with the regularity of phonation, and may also affect segmental contrasts, but in this example normal rhythm and intonation contrasts are preserved.

3. This speaker habitually uses an extended pitch range, with exaggerated intonation patterns which listeners may interpret as implying much stronger emotion than the speaker intends, since wide pitch movements convey an intensification of attitude in NAS English.

4. Unusually high, narrow pitch range. Intonation contrasts are intact and rhythm is normal, but this speaker may unintentionally convey lack of interest because of the range restriction, and/or lack of maturity because of high pitch.

It should be noted that while one example of each type is sufficient to illustrate the point, many more are required to enable abstraction of a particular system from a speech sample. In addition, the overlapping effects of different segmental and non-segmental systems may obfuscate the particular aspect concerned, necessitating careful elicitation of appropriate material as a basis for analysis where this is the case.

"I think they're on the chair. No... under the chair."

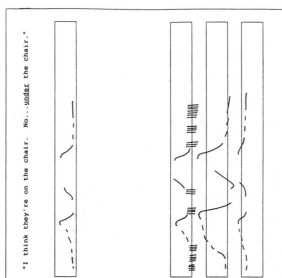

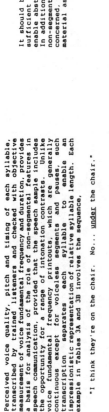

Figure 4.1 Some intonation patterns produced by deaf speakers

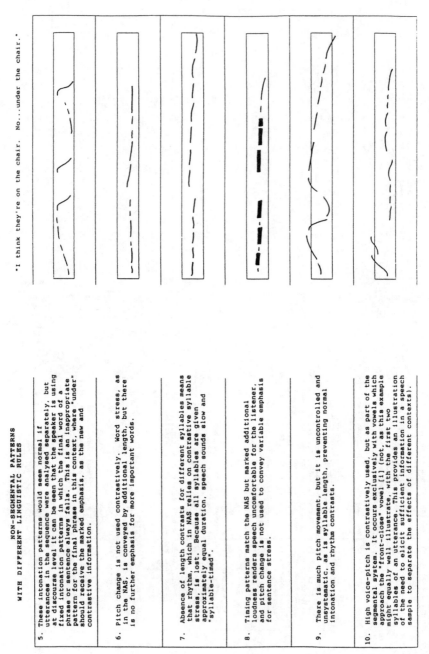

"I think they're on the chair.   No...under the chair."

**NON-SEGMENTAL PATTERNS
WITH DIFFERENT LINGUISTIC RULES**

5. These intonation patterns would seem normal if utterances in the sequence were analysed separately, but at discourse level it can be seen that the speaker is using fixed intonation patterns in which the final word of a phrase or sentence always falls. This is an inappropriate pattern for the final phrase in this context, where "under" should receive the marked emphasis, as the new and contrastive information.

6. Pitch change is not used contrastively. Word stress, as in the NAS, is conveyed by additional length, but there is no further emphasis for more important words.

7. Absence of length contrasts for different syllables means that rhythm, which in NAS relies on contrastive syllable stress, is lost. Because all syllables are given approximately equal duration, speech sounds slow and "syllable-timed".

8. Timing patterns match the NAS but marked additional loudness renders speech uncomfortable for the listener, and pitch change is not used to convey variable emphasis for sentence stress.

9. There is much pitch movement, but it is uncontrolled and unsystematic, as is syllable length, preventing normal intonation and rhythm contrasts.

10. High voice-pitch is contrastively used, but as part of the segmental system. It occurs exclusively with vowels which approach the "front-close" vowel [i] (not this example might equally well illustrate, with the first syllables of an utterance. Thus provides an illustration of the need to elicit sufficient information in a speech sample to separate the effects of different contexts).

Figure 4.1 contd.

speech intelligibility to different interlocutors, rather than seeking to dismiss it.

An attempt to account for the speaker's system in both auditory (audible) and visual terms would seem particularly relevant in terms of the underlying perceptual basis—a difference in hearing—for the observed differences from the adult, normal speech sound system.

If such an attempt is made, the speech of deaf people seems to fall naturally into a range of pattern-types, which relate somewhat closely to (overlapping) ranges of intelligibility for different interlocutors, which can be described without recourse to the unhelpful notion of speech 'errors'. This offers a comparatively simple framework for assessment. Such a framework is presented in Table 4.2 and, at this point, a further circularity needs to be interrupted for the sake of clarity. The speaker types in the proposed categories were reached after a protracted exercise of narrow transcription and inter-transcriber comparison, in a survey of the speech of 71 deaf adults (Irlam, 1982) and in a longer term, continuing project on assessment, transcription and measurement. However, if the suggested categories are used as the initial basis for speech assessment, as well as a summarising end-point, the need for protracted transcription of individual speakers can be reduced, by means of a 'probe-test' to indicate the category, followed by a detailed assessment procedure if necessary. In two of the categories (Speaker Types 1 and 5) for different reasons, detailed transcription may be neither necessary nor appropriate.

Table 4.2 Types of pattern, listeners and speech intelligibility

---

Type 1 Phonetic-level differences from NAS

Phonetic differences in vowels, consonants, timing and intonation: slight or marked. No reductions in linguistic contrasts: NAS minimal pairs, such as 'sun/ton', still distinguishable. Speakers intelligible to most listeners, however, inexperienced, unless in high noise levels.

Type 2 Phonetic and phonological differences

Quality may sound similar to Type 1 speakers, but phonetic changes involve reduction in phonological contrasts: NAS minimal pairs, such as 'sun/ton', sound identical. Speech therefore more difficult to understand than for Type 1, especially in challenging conditions (public speaking, poor acoustic environment).

Type 3 Consistent visual system

Linguistic contrasts more severely reduced, and mainly based on visual contrasts (visible place of articulation). Auditory features (manner and voicing of speech segments, voice quality and intonation) absent or restricted: thus 'sun/ton' may be indistinguishable from each other and from a range of other similar words.

Table 4.2 Contd.

Speech intelligible to experienced listenders who lipread and use contextual redundancy. Use of additional cues (such as finger-spelling or signs from BSL) may help visual intelligibility. Inexperienced listeners have much more difficulty.

Type 4 Inconsistent visual system

Severe system reduction. Visual basis as for Type 3, but much variability of audible features (such as airstream mechanism, voicing, manner of articulation, intonation, timing) makes 'tuning in' more difficult. Words, such as 'sun/ton' not contrasted with each other, and vary from one instance to another. Intelligibility range: high (for experienced listener using cues as for Type 3) to very low (inexperienced listener relying on auditory contrasts).

Type 5 BSL preferred: spoken language minimal

Speakers from Types 1–4 above may be bilingual (in spoken languages, or spoken language and sign language). For this group, sign language is the first and preferred language, minimal use of spoken English being used when necessary to communicate with monolingual speech users. The 'speaker' has a full and adequate other language as the basis of communication, and *speech* assessment would completely miss the point.

Many speakers who are deaf have characteristic voice and speech patterns, which are different from most hearing speakers of the same dialect, and which may render the speaker recognisable as an individual with a hearing loss, although he or she is for the most part highly intelligible. For these speakers (Type 1; the 'most intelligible to most listeners' group) speech patterns are usually adequately described in terms of overall articulatory 'settings' (see Chapter 3), and any differences from the general pattern will for many speakers be readily observable, by the phonetically trained listener, from a relatively brief and unstructured spontaneous speech sample. 'Error analysis' is as inappropriate for this group of speakers as for any other, because, although it is possible that all the speech sounds and all the non-segmental features are somewhat different phonetically from normal adult speech, they are not different enough to be confusable one with another (the full system of segmental and non-segmental linguistic contrasts is preserved). Thus error analysis may produce 'all errors' or 'no errors' for the same speaker, dependant on what the listener is prepared to accept as 'normal', but such results will not explain what is happening in the speech, or why it is so intelligible to most people, or why it is sometimes difficult to understand. A phonetic description of the overall articulatory settings and acoustic results for speech production is a more powerful and revealing way to explain the patterns observed for this group of speakers.

For another group (Type 5), any attempt to analyse speech patterns at phonetic and phonological levels alone would be irrelevant, since speech is not the language concerned, even for those members of the group who are bilingual in sign language and written English. It is true that individuals in this group may use some spoken language forms when necessary, and that analysis of such speech production might show a severely reduced and simplified phonological system, but in this context any attempt to describe communication simply in terms of the speech-sound patterns that might be elicited by a formal speech assessment would completely miss the point.

It is the three other groups in Table 4.2, Types 2–4 for whom the careful elicitation of a structured speech sample seems most important, if an accurate analysis of patterns is to form the basis for intervention. Superficially, the three speaker types may seem similar, and traditional error-counts may not reveal the highly specific types of pattern which differentiate the groups. Analysis of the contrastive phonology used by speakers produces these three distinctive pattern-types:

1. A full set of phonological contrasts even though phonetic realisations may be different from the NAS (Type 2).
2. A reduced set of contrasts which matches the visible range of contrasts of the spoken language, lacks audible contrasts but is highly consistent (Type 3).
3. An inconsistent system with many audible features in free variation, which makes 'tuning in' to the system which exists more difficult (Type 4).

Any of these speakers may, of course, be bilingual in sign and spoken language (for example, BSL and English in the UK) and 'interlanguage' features may support speech intelligibility, as may the previous experience and skills of the listener. There is therefore not a simple relationship of the speaker-types described with speech intelligibility.

In both transcription and analysis, the relevance of the visual as well as the auditory mode needs to be considered in a number of ways. Firstly, in spoken language visual cues may supplement or supplant the auditory signal, so that speech intelligibility is enhanced for the 'listener' who lipreads (and therefore perceives silent articulatory gestures, and other information which is visually mapped on to the NAS, as part of the accessible speech signal). Secondly, use of additional visible cues, such as fingerspelling or simultaneous signing, may further disambiguate the signal for the listener who understands the cues. In this way, speakers whose phonology, in auditory terms, is highly inconsistent and difficult for inexperienced listeners to understand (Type 4) or even non-existent (in the case of speakers who use no voice at all but nevertheless communicate in English) may be 100% intelligible to an experienced 'speechreader'.

Thirdly, if intervention to improve speech intelligibility is considered, a vital question may be, 'intelligibility to whom?'. If the speaker wishes to be more intelligible to strangers, then it may be most relevant to focus on the audible phonology and general tactics for effective communication, with the emphasis on extending the speech and communicative skills of the speaker. If, on the other hand, the individual is more concerned with communication with family and friends, then visible aspects of communication, and the ability of the family and friends to use them, may be as important as the speech of the speaker. In the case of deafened adults, new communicative skills may be needed by both speaker and listener.

Finally, if this type of account addresses both the linguistic system and the phonetic realisations, both the segmental phonology and the non-segmental systems, and if an adequate sample of speech and is elicited for the purpose, the apparent complexity of speech assessment can be broken down into a comparatively simple frame of reference, such as the speech category system presented in Table 4.2. The complexity lies in the preparatory work—the audio-visual training of the assessor, the linguistic understanding required to produce a phonological analysis, and the acquisition of adequate personal communication skills to enable a hearing person to work with deaf people as clients and as colleagues. When this hard work has been undertaken, the assessment of a deaf individual's speech is not a complex issue, although the continuing controversy about the status of 'speech' for the deaf community may well provide a more than compensatory challenge.

Acknowledgements

Part of the work on which this chapter was based was supported by a North East Thames Regional Health Authority Grant, and we should particularly like to thank our colleagues at University College Hospital, London, Enid Wechsler and the late Graham Fraser, who were closely involved with the original project. In addition, a number of other colleagues have given support and advice, and we are especially grateful to Robert Fawcus of City University, Mike Martin of the Royal National Institute for Deaf People, Lena Rustin of Camden and Islington Health Authorities, and John Weinman of Guy's Hospital, London.

Appendix

Examples of transcriptions of deaf speakers: the need for accurate observation

Target and transcription

cat [Kxæ(t)]   table [dɛɪ(bəl)]

Notes

Silent articulations (of the syllable-final consonant in 'cat' and the second syllable of 'table' will be inaccessible to the transcriber of an audio-tape recording, but a correct speech analysis and appropriate intervention may depend on the recognition of such features. The pattern to be identified in analysis is not *omission* of final consonant or final syllable, but non-sustension of airstream and/or voicing, leading to a partial (visual) realisation of final syllables and syllable-final consonants.

Target and transcription

tea [t3]   two [t3]

Notes

Auditorily, the two vowels in this NAS minimal pair are identical segments which would be indistinguishable on an audiotape recording. An experienced transcriber who includes visible features will be able to explain why the two words (and the vowel system in general) are not confused by listeners who know this speaker, since they are able to lipread the difference conveyed by contrastive lipspreading and liprounding, although there is no consistent auditory effect. An untrained observer might not be able to separate the contrast as 'correct' (which it is visually) or mark it 'absent' (which it is auditorily). To capture the phonetic basis of this speaker's intelligibility to known interlocutors and difficulty in communication with strangers (and to provide helpful intervention if necessary) requires accurate observation of both visual and auditory components.

Target and transcription

Ben [bɛn]   pen [bɛn]   men [ᵥbɛn]

Notes

To the trained and experienced observer, the difference between implosive/voiced/prevoiced bilabial consonants provides a detectable basis for this speaker's highly intelligible equivalent to the NAS voiced/voiceless/nasal contrast. Incorrect transcription or error analysis could result in focus on the 'incorrect' realisations rather than the intact phonological level, which involves consistent linguistic contrast. Intervention to 'correct' the most 'distorted' sound (the implosive) to [b] would reduce the system of contrasts.

Target and transcription

The man was fat	[dʒ ban wɒ baʔ]
	man *fat*
The man was Pat	[dʒ ban wɒ baʔ]
	man PAT

Notes

Transcription only of the spoken elements (upper elements of the transcription) shows the ambiguity of the utterance for the inexperienced listener, but misses the intelligibility provided (without any other contextual information) for the experienced listener by simultaneous sign (*fat*) and fingerspelling (PAT).

References

Bamford, J. and Saunders, E. (1982) *Hearing Impairment, Auditory Perception and Language Disability* (2nd edition). London, Edward Arnold

Bouvet, D. (1990) *The Path to Language: Bilingual Education for Deaf Children.* Clevedon: Multilingual Matters

Brentari, D.K. and Wolk, S. (1986) The relative effects of three expressive methods upon the speech intelligibility of profoundly deaf speakers. *Journal of Communication Disorders,* 19 (3), 209—218

Catford, J.C. (1988) *A Practical Introduction to Phonetics.* Oxford: Clarenden Press

Connor, L.E. (Ed.). (1971) *Speech of the Deaf Child.* Washington D.C.: Alexander Graham Bell Association

Couper-Kuhlen, E. (1986) *An Introduction to English Prosody.* London: Edward Arnold

Crystal, D. (1987) *Clinical Linguistics* (2nd edition). London: Edward Arnold

Deuchar, M. (1984) *British Sign Language.* London: Routledge & Kegan Paul

Duckworth, M., Allen, G., Hardcastle, W. and Ball, M. (1990) Extensions to the International Phonetic Alphabet for the transcription of atypical speech. *Clinical Linguistics and Phonetics* 4.4, 273—280

Finkelstein, V. (1984) 'We' are not disabled, 'you' are. In: Gregory, S. and Hartly, G. (eds). *Constructing Deafness*. Milton Keynes: Open University Press

Fletcher, L. (1983) *A Language for Ben*. London: Souvenir Press

Gimson, A.C. (1989) *An Introduction to the Pronunciation of English* (2nd edition, revised by Susan Ramsaran). London: Edward Arnold

Green, K. and Rees, R. (1992) Intervention with deaf children requires a pragmatic approach. *Human Communication*, May issue

Gregory, S. and Hartly. G. (1984) *Constructing Deafness*. Milton Keynes: Open University Press

Gregory, S. and Mogford, K. (1981) Early language development. In: Deuchar, M., Kyle, J. and Woll, B. (eds). *Perspectives on British Sign Language and Deafness*. London: Croom Helm

Grosjean, F. (1982) *Life with Two Languages: An Introduction to Bilingualism*. Cambridge, M.A.: Harvard University Press

Grunwell, P. (1987) *Clinical Phonology* (2nd edition). London: Croom Helm

Gudykunst, E. (Ed.) (1988) *Language and Ethnic Indentity*. Clevedon: Multilingual Matters

Halden, J. and Gaughan, R. (1986) A specialist service for individual needs. *Speech Therapy in Practice* (September issue)

Hochberg, I., Levitt, H. and Osberger, M.J. (1983) *Speech of the Hearing Impaired*, Baltimore: University Park Press

Horii, Y. (1982) Some voice fundamental frequency characteristics of oral reading and spontaneous speech by hard-of-hearing young women. *Journal of Speech and Hearing Research*, 25, 608–610

Irlam, S. (1982) The speech of hearing-impaired adults and some results of speech therapy. University of London: unpublished M.Sc. dissertation

Johns-Lewis, C. (Ed.). (1986) *Intonation in Discourse*. London: Croom Helm

Kelly, J. and Local, J. (1989) *Doing Phonology: Observing, Recording, Interpreting*. Manchester: Manchester University Press

Kyle, J.G. (Ed.). (1987) *Adjustment to Acquired Hearing Loss: Analysis, Change and Learning*. Bristol: Bristol Centre for Deaf Studies, University of Bristol

Kyle, J.G. and Woll, B. (1985) *Sign Language: The Study of Deaf People and Their Language*. Cambridge: Cambridge University Press

Ladd, D.R. (1980) *The Structure of Intonational Meaning: Evidence from English*. Bloomington: Indiana University Press

Lane, H. (Ed.). (1984a) *The Deaf Experience*. Cambridge, M.A.: Harvard University Press

Lane, H. (1984b) *When the Mind Hears*. London: Pelican

Levitt, H. and Stromberg, H. (1983) Segmental characteristics of the speech of hearing-impaired children: factors affecting intelligibility. In: Hochberg, I., Levitt, H. and Osberger, M.J. *Speech of the Hearing Impaired*. Baltimore: University Park Press

Ling, D. (1976) *Speech and the Hearing Impaired Child: Theory and Practice*. Washington, D.C.: Alexander Graham Bell Association

Llewellyn-Jones, M. and Wirt, A. (1988) Assessing communication in a bilingual setting. Paper presented at the Second Conference of the British Association of Teachers of the Deaf and the College of Speech Therapists, Birmingham.

Lysons, K. (1984) *Hearing Impairment: A Guide to People with Auditory Handicaps and Those Concerned with their Care and Rehabilitation*. London: Woodhead Faulkner Ltd

Markides, A. (1983) *The Speech of Hearing Impaired Children*. Manchester: Manchester University Press

Meadow, K.P. (1980) *Deafness and Child Development*. London: Edward Arnold

Mindel, E.D. and McCay, V. (1987) *They Grow in Silence*. Massachusetts: College Hill Press

Mulholland, A.M. (1981) *Oral Education Today and Tomorrow*. Washington, D.C.: Alexander Graham Bell Association

National Aural Group (NAG) (1981) Promoting natural language through residual hearing. *Journal of the British Association of Teachers of the Deaf*, **5**, (3), 8–11

National Deaf Children's Society (NDCS) (1987) *Always a Step Behind: Children with Acquired Deafness*, London: NDSC

Nittrouer, S. and Hocherg, I. (1985) Speech instruction for deaf children: a communication-based approach. *American Annals of the Deaf*, December issue

Osberger, M. and Levitt, H. (1979) The effect of timing errors on the intelligibility of deaf children's speech. *Journal of the Acoustical Society of America*, **66**, 1316–1324

Padden, C.P. and Humphries, T. (1988) *Deaf in America: Voices from a Culture*. Cambridge, M.A.: Harvard University Press

Parker, A. and Rose, H. (1990) Deaf children's phonological development. In: Grunwell, P. (Ed.). *Developmental Speech Disorders*. London: Churchill Livingstone

Parker, A. and Wirz, S. (1986). Towards a better understanding: speech therapy with deaf people. *Speech Therapy in Practice* (September issue)

PRDS Group (1980) *The phonetic representation of disordered speech*. British Journal of Disorders of Communication, **15**, 217–223

Pring, T.R. (1986) Evaluating the effects of speech therapy for aphasics: developing a single case methodology. *British Journal of Disorders of Communication*, **21**, 1, 103–116

Pye, C., Wilcox, K.A. and Siren, K. (1988) Refining transcriptions: the significance of transcriber 'errors'. *Journal of Child Language*, **15**, 17–37.

Quigley, S.P. and Paul, P.D. (1984) *Language and Deafness*. San Diego: College Hill Press

Sacks, O. (1991) *Seeing Voices*. London: Pan Books

Sainsbury, S. (1986) *Deaf Worlds*, London: Heinemann

Schlesinger, H. (1978) The acquisition of bimodal language. In: Schlesinger, H. and Namir, L. (eds). *Sign Language of the Deaf: International Perspectives*. New York: Academic Press

Schlesinger, H. and Namir, L. (eds). *Sign Language of the Deaf: International Perspectives*. New York: Academic Press

Stathopoulos, E.T., Duchan, J.F., Sonnenmeier, R.M. and Bruce, N.V. (1986) Intonation and pausing in deaf speech. *Folia Phoniatrica*, **38**, 1–12

Stevens, K.N., Nickerson, R.S. and Rollins, A.M. (1983) Suprasegmental and postural aspects of speech production and their effect on articulatory skills and intelligibility. In: Hochberg, I., Levitt, H. and Osberger, M.J. (eds). *The Speech of the Hearing Impaired*. Baltimore: University Park Press

Stoel-Gammon, C. (1983) The acquisition of segmental phonology by normal and hearing-impaired children. In: Hochberg, I., Levitt, H. and Osberger, M.J. (eds). *Speech of the Hearing Impaired*. Baltimore: University Park Press

Summerfield, Q. (1983) Audiovisual speech perception, lipreading and artificial stimulation. In: Lutman, M. and Haggard, M. (eds). *Hearing Science and Hearing Disorders*. London: Academic Press

Taylor, G. and Bishop, J. (1991) *Being Deaf: The Experience of Deafness*. Milton

Keynes: Open University Press

Watts, W.J. (Ed.). (1983) *Rehabilitation and Acquired Deafness*. London: Croom Helm

Whitehead, R.L. (1983) Some respiratory and aerodynamic patterns in the speech of the hearing impaired. In: Hochberg, I., Levitt, H. and Osberger, M.J. (eds) *Speech of the Hearing Impaired*. Baltimore: University Park Press

Wilcox, S. (Ed.) (1988) *American Deaf Culture: An Anthology* T&J Publishers

Woll., B. and Lawson, L. (1980) British Sign Language. In: Bristol University School of Education Research Unit. *Research on Deafness and BSL*. London: RNID

Woll, B., Kyle, J.G., and Deuchar, M. (1981) *Perspectives on BSL and Deafness*. London: Croom Helm

Wood, D.J., Wood, H.A., Griffiths, A.J. and Howarth, C.I. (1986) *Teaching and Talking with Deaf Children*. London: Wiley

Woodward, (1982) *On Depathologising Deafness*. T&J Publishers

Chapter 5
Perceptual assessment in aphasia

Elizabeth Dean and Christine Skinner

Introduction

The rationale for the use of perceptual analysis incorporates many points that have valuable implications for the description and remediation of the aphasic condition. Most aphasiologists recognise the need to examine not only language breakdown but also communicative strength. However, the criticism often levelled at perceptive analysis is that assessment of communication function lacks rigour. This chapter will attempt to illustrate that this assertion is false by drawing on the literature relating to the assessment and remediation of communicative functioning.

Green (1984) provides a concise description of perceptual analysis:

> The assessment relies upon auditory perception. The ear of the therapist is, in the final analysis, the most telling evaluation possible (p. 37).

When applied to aphasiology we can paraphrase this citation to read:

> The assessment relies upon the perception of communicative strength. The eyes and ears of the therapist are, in the final analysis, the most telling evaluation possible.

This paraphrase encapsulates the argument explored in this chapter: that assessment of aphasia must not merely record the completeness of the spoken and written output of the aphasic person but also must consider the totality of the communicative performance. To do this the analyst/assessor has to respond as an interactive partner with the aphasic person rather than adopting the role of an observer.

This chapter will present two strands of evidence which highlight the importance of perceptual assessment with aphasic people. First, evidence that assessment which only focuses on analysis of spoken and written language processing will give an incomplete picture of communicative functioning. Second, there is evidence that different aspects of communicative performance may respond differentially to the initial trauma and/or the remediation process. Having presented the evidence the chapter will go on to consider the range of attempts which have been made to capture the elusive nature of communicative functioning and will then focus on one such profile, the *Revised Edinburgh Functional Communication Profile* (REFCP), (Wirz, Skinner and Dean, 1990), as a basis for discussion of the issues which still remain to be resolved.

The nature of communicative functioning and its implications for aphasiology

In 1969 Sarno published the *Functional Communication Profile* and in doing so provided the focus for a new movement within aphasiology which recognised the importance of the relationship between linguistic performance and communicative ability. In 1977 Holland made the comment that has now become so well known: 'aphasics probably communicate better than they talk' (p. 173). Currently, there is increasing evidence that assessment which focuses solely on linguistic performance is insufficient (see, for example, Gurland, Chwat and Wollner, 1982; Holland, 1982; Behrman and Penn, 1984; Green, 1984; Davis and Wilcox, 1985; Simmons, 1986; Penn, 1988; Herrmann et al., 1989). What are the grounds for this increasing dissatisfaction with formal assessments of linguistic functioning? Objective testing to determine the nature and extent of language processing difficulties is obviously a prerequisite for the construction and re-evaluation of a principled management programme. However, there is a growing awareness that, to be comprehensive, the assessment process must also take account, first, of the aphasic person's use of communicative modalities, such as gesture, facial expression and intonation, and, second, of the context in which communication takes place.

This wider view is vital for several reasons. There is evidence that different communicative modalities may be differentially affected by the initial trauma and, once disrupted, may respond differentially to the remediation process. Further, there is strong clinical evidence that the processing of disordered communication may be even more responsive than the normal communicative process to the effect of context. Thus, failure by the therapist to appreciate the value of manipulating the context of the interaction will lead to assessment and remediation being less than useful.

The role of context and its implications for assessment

Attempts to supplement assessment of linguistic functioning have increasingly drawn upon pragmatic theory; this is a diverse field but one which has been of growing interest in academic linguistics since the 1970s. Pragmatics was defined by Bate (1982) as:

> ... the study of language in context. It looks at how words are used to inter-act with and influence people. The pragmatics of language is language in use — what people do with words and how they adapt what they say to the needs of differing listeners and situations (p. 17).

In 1987 Prutting and Kirchner described pragmatics as being concerned with 'the relationship between linguistic knowledge and the principles governing language use'. The common thread between the many definitions of pragmatics is that *communication* occurs in *context*. For an interaction to be fully understood it is necessary not only to consider the syntax and semantics but also to take account of the context in which the discourse occurs. In their protocol Prutting and Kirchner (1987) provide a framework for observing pragmatic functioning in three areas: verbal aspects, paralinguistic aspects, and non-verbal aspects. Davis and Wilcox (1985) suggest that, in general, aphasic clients retain pragmatic skills such as those detailed in the *Pragmatic Protocol* of Prutting and Kirchner. Other researchers have provided evidence within specific areas of communication and context.

In an observational study Holland (1982) recorded the communication skills of 40 dysphasic people. She concluded that aphasic clients had some primitive but useful functional solutions to their communication problems. That is, that they had a surprisingly wide range of successful communicative acts despite the fact that their utterances were linguistically disordered. In this study, the most communicative dysphasic people did not differ in their use of successful communication acts from non-aphasic speakers observed over a similar period of time. The only difference was that the successful communication of the latter contained a higher proportion of 'well formed' utterances.

Several authors have reported that aphasic speakers successfully use a range of speech acts, such as greeting, questioning, requesting, stating, and negating. Prinz (1980), for example, focusing on the production of requests, concluded that regardless of the type or severity of the aphasia, his subjects appeared capable of formulating requests utilising both verbal and non-verbal strategies. The influence of the degree of communicative deficit was seen in the type of strategy utilised; the global aphasic clients tended to rely more on gestural and contextual information to convey meaning, whereas the client with Broca's aphasia depended more on verbal strategies.

Traditional assessments for aphasic clients do not focus on the ability of the individual to convey meaning but almost invariably on the ability to perform specific tasks. Although such procedures have the advantage of presenting a standard test situation which can be replicated easily, failure to take account of the broader ability to perform a range of speech acts, to convey different meaning, will lead to much valuable information being disregarded.

Further, the influence of the context within which communication takes place upon the expressive and receptive abilities of aphasic people has also been addressed in the literature (see for example: Green, 1984; Davis and Wilcox, 1985; Karilahti, 1987; Lesser and Milroy, 1987; Davis, 1989) but has rarely been explicitly studied. The majority of formal assessments of aphasia try to reduce the influence of context to a minimum in their attempts to seek objectivity. This process has the advantage of standardisation but the disadvantage of becoming an 'exercise' far removed from communication. An utterance does not occur, nor is it interpreted, in isolation. A familiar situation will increase the likelihood that a sentence with a complex syntactic structure will be understood by the aphasic client. Similarly, 'background' knowledge that the speaker and listener share will contribute to an aphasic utterance being comprehended. The communicative environment can be manipulated to enhance the aphasic person's functioning, and to minimise the effect of the language disorder. As remediation is directed towards improving performance in 'normal' communicative settings, assessment which does not provide information pertinent to this is limited. It is the argument of this chapter that when the therapist profiles the communicative performance of clients (in addition to results from standardised assessments) there will be a more balanced base from which to plan remediation.

The role of context and its implications for remediation

Traditionally, aphasia therapy has used tasks which 'train specific linguistic elements' (Green, 1984). This may be a valuable medium within which to facilitate spoken or written language but the essential value of language, that it facilitates interaction between individuals, must not be ignored. Increasingly during the last decade the literature has focused on the need to ground specific linguistic tasks within the framework of natural communication.

There are two main reasons for this. The first arises from the insights provided by work describing the influence of context on communication. Spoken and written language will be facilitated by manipulation of the communicative context. An example of a remediation programme which capitalises on this is PACE therapy (Davis and Wilcox, 1981; 1985). Here, the quality and quantity of information conveyed by an aphasic person within a conversation are maximised by the fact that the activity requires new information to be passed to the listener. This is in contrast to much traditional therapy where the therapist aims to reduce the chances that the aphasic person will fail to get his message across by asking only for known information. If the aphasic person is aware of this, as indeed would be the case if both were looking at the picture to be described, output may be reduced because of the assumption of shared knowledge. This example illustrates the way in which context can be altered to maximise language use.

A very different example centres on management of the aphasic problem not by direct intervention with the client but by working with care-givers. It might be possible to enhance a client's potential to comprehend not by therapy but by giving advice to care-givers about, for example, the type of input the aphasic person is likely to understand (Gravel and LaPointe, 1982; Brumfitt and Clarke 1983; Green, 1984).

The considerable current interest in pragmatics within aphasiology arises from its appeal for clinicians who have long been concerned that a focus on narrowly defined linguistic competences is a restricted basis for the management of aphasic clients. If aphasia therapy can be set within the context of *language in use* its efficacy will be enhanced and the learning more readily generalised to situations outside the clinic. In addition, an emphasis on communicative competence can permit social reintegration for aphasic people for whom linguistic accuracy will never be a possibility. There is now a need for sustained research to objectify the study of clinical communication by isolating relevant and measurable parameters. Current developments in the field of profiling language performance will be explored later in this chapter.

The role of communicative modalities and their implications for assessment

The studies by Holland (1982) and Prinz (1980) cited above illustrate a further vital factor about communication which is not addressed in formal assessments of language processing. In both these studies the subjects conveyed different communicative functions by utilising alternative modalities. The interaction did not necessarily take place within the media of spoken and/or written language, the modalities which generally form the focus of aphasia tests. A series of other papers have provided support for the argument that non-verbal performance should be profiled in aphasia assessments. Some of these studies have purported to show that aphasic people can acquire, and do use, some type of non-verbal system, or spontaneous non-verbal behaviours, for communication, to a degree which is significantly greater than their processing of spoken and/or written language (for example, Schlanger and Freimann, 1979; Skelly, 1979; Helm-Estabrooks, Fitzpatrick and Barresti, 1981; Herrmann et al., 1988).

Such findings not only have obvious implications for the development of management programmes but also provide insights into the very nature of aphasia. The ability of aphasic people to communicate non-verbally has been taken as an argument against there being a central cognitive/symbolic deficit, such as that proposed by Finkelberg (Duffy and Liles, 1979) who argued that aphasia should more accurately be termed 'asymbolia'. At a basic level the debate concerns the nature of the disruption to the cognitive operations underlying language. Supporting evidence for the competing hypotheses has been gathered from studies of the ability of aphasic people to process non-verbal symbol systems, such as gesture, facial expression, tactile symbols and written symbols. (A comprehensive review of earlier studies is provided by Feyereisen and Seron, 1982a, 1982b).

Unfortunately, the overriding characteristic of many studies of non-verbal communication and aphasia is the wide range of ability that the subjects demonstrate. Forming hypotheses about the reason for this diversity is hindered by the fact that in many of these papers subject variables, such as type of aphasia, time post-onset, and cognitive ability are not used as controlled, independent experimental variables and concomitant difficulties, such as motor processing limitations are loosely defined and poorly measured.

A paper by Le May, David and Thomas (1988) illustrates a current extension of the 'asymbolia' question which does have potentially useful clinical implications. The study of Le May et al. (1988) was designed to investigate the use of gesture in a group of clients suffering from Wernicke's aphasia, Broca's aphasia, and non-neurologically impaired comparison subjects. The results indicated that aphasic subjects used more spontaneous gesture than controls and that the frequency and type of gesture differed according to the type of aphasia. Those with Broca's aphasia used more gesture than those with Wernicke's aphasia. Le May et al. (1988) conclude that when aphasic clients are faced with verbal communication difficulties they will compensate by using more gesture. This finding, they argue, supports the hypothesis that both speech and gesture are 'governed' by a central organiser but can function independently to compensate for verbal impairments.

In a study with a slightly different emphasis, Ferro et al. (1980) compared recovery trends in clients with Broca's and Wernicke's aphasia and found that non-verbal abilities improved more than verbal language and that improvement in the interpretation of gesture was correlated positively with oral comprehension recovery, in particular for those with Wernicke's aphasia. This study points to one of the major objects of assessment, the formation of a baseline for management programmes. One of the strongest arguments for taking account of the effect of a range of communicative modalities and the communicative context is their relevance to intervention.

The role of communicative modalities and their implications for remediation

The argument for grounding therapy within a communicative framework is based on the notion that at certain points in the remediation process the therapist should concentrate on maximising communicative potential by use of any available modality rather than focusing specifically on the accuracy of spoken or written language. Although the importance of assessing and treating communicative ability rather than language skills is increasingly recognised by clinicians the approach has not been studied as extensively, or as systematically, as other approaches, such as cognitive neuropsychology.

Examples of published therapy programmes which focus on communicative competence include *Functional Communication Therapy* (Aten, Caliguiri and Holland, 1982), PACE (Davis and Wilcox, 1985), *Total Communication Therapy* (Dean, Skinner and Edmonson, 1987) and several case studies (for example, Green, 1982; Edelman, 1983; Parsons et al., 1989). In the main, the thrust of these therapeutic programmes has been to capitalise on communicative abilities which have not been disrupted as much as verbal language skills.

The findings of these studies are hard to evaluate. In addition to methodological difficulties outlined above, the variation in ability displayed by different subjects, contribute to the enormous difficulties inherent in trying to devise a valid, reliable and clinically useful measure of communication. The results of studies, such as those of Aten, Caligiuri and Holland (1982) and Davis and Wilcox (1985) have been encouraging. However, the complexity of the issues involved is becoming clear. For example, Dean, Skinner and Edmonson (1987) reported a small-scale study of the effect of *Total Communication Therapy* with a group of five long-term aphasic people living in a long stay hospital. The authors found that the intervention did not produce significant change on assessments of communicative functioning, despite positive reports by ward staff, but did produce shifts in the aphasia quotients as measured by a standardised aphasia test. The authors concluded that this set of single case studies raised a series of questions about issues such as the sensitivity of current assessments of communicative functioning, despite the fact that change was noted by ward staff and therapists.

These inconclusive results can perhaps best be explained by suggesting that it is the specific nature of the linguistic impairment which determines how successful an aphasic person will be by use of an alternative or augmentative system. In a recent study Wirz, Dean and Benham (1989) found that those aphasic subjects judged to be the most 'efficient' communicators were those who retained relatively good semantic processing abilities. Alternative and augmentative systems of communication may function optimally for aphasic clients who have relatively intact semantic processing but impairments at the level of the input and/or output lexicons.

Similarly, Le May et al. (1988) conclude that their results did not 'support the pessimistic opinion that conceptual or motor deficits prevent the use of gesture by aphasic subjects to convey precise meanings' (p. 29) and argue that the facilitation of the gestural mode may be a fruitful therapeutic aim but that aphasic people with different language processing impairments will require different therapeutic regimes to achieve the aim of augmenting verbal with gestural communication.

Such conclusions have relevance for the interpretation of earlier studies of the extent to which aphasic people can learn more formal gestural systems, (Schlanger and Freimann, 1979; Skelly, 1979; Helm-Estabrooks, Fitzpatrick and Barresti, 1981; Coelho and Duffy, 1987). It can be hypothesised that the aphasic person's success, or otherwise depended upon the level(s) at which his language processing was disrupted and the severity of the impairment.

The literature that has been reviewed in this chapter provides evidence of the value of including gestural techniques in the treatment of aphasia. The clinician working with an aphasic person observes discrepancies between measurements of his abilities, by use of standard assessments or batteries, and the communicative successes when the same client wants to share information important to him. However, more and more precise studies are required if the relationship between the competences underlying verbal and non-verbal processing is to be fully understood and exploited.

The assessment of communicative function

Emphasis on function as well as structure of language has forced aphasiologists to consider the powerful influence of context on communication and the extent to which aphasic speakers are able to rely on their pragmatic knowledge in communicative interaction. This demands a flexibility by therapists in assessment and, subsequently, treatment methods to ensure that they measure not only how accurately but also how successfully an aphasic person communicates a message. The measurement of communicative success is achieved by observation and the use of assessment materials.

The major goals of functional communication assessment are detailed by Simmons (1986) as follows: to add information needed for differential diagnosis; assist in focusing treatment; provide in-depth information on relative communication strengths and weaknesses for specific modalities in order to assist in management and counselling;

and to provide more sensitive measures of behavioural change over time. This latter goal has proved to be the most difficult to achieve; lack of sensitivity and objectivity have been the main criticisms of this perceptual assessment.

Recent advances aim to address this issue by developing more rigorous and systematic identification and isolation of the rather heterogeneous range of abilities which make up communicative effectiveness (Lesser and Milroy, 1987). The clinician who seeks some published structure for the assessment of the communicative effectiveness of aphasic people has available six published procedures: Sarno (1969); Wilcox and Davis (1977); Prutting (1982); Penn (1983); Skinner et al. (1984); and Wirz, Skinner and Dean (1990). The authors argue that the latter, the REFCP (Wirz, Skinner and Dean, 1990) addresses the interactive nature of the communicative effectiveness between aphasic and non-aphasic people more fully than the others.

As long ago as 1969, Sarno, with the introducion of the *Functional Communication Profile* (Sarno 1969) criticised traditional aphasia tests for being measures of potential rather than actual language use. She maintained that standard practice in the language evaluation of aphasia measured clinical performance and not the unforced, voluntary and habitual utterances which characterise normal spoken language. In an attempt to answer these criticisms, the *Functional Communication Profile* (FCP) was designed to quantify the communication behaviours which a client actually uses in the course of interaction with others, regardless of severity of impairment. Wilcox and Davis (1977) analysed aphasic communication in terms of impairment of specific speech acts in order to sample the ability of the aphasic person to communicate a variety of intentions. Based on the concepts of Searle (1969), Wilcox and Davis (1977) classified speech acts into such categories as 'requests', 'assertions' and 'questions'. Interestingly, speech-act analysis revealed that during treatment clinicians predominantly used the speech acts of questions and requests, whereas patients responded with a predominance of assertions. The investigators observed that traditional therapy might actually restrict the range of speech acts a patient uses, resulting in dependence on others for the initiation of conversation. Speech-act analysis, therefore, appears to hold useful principles upon which to create situations that require communication of a variety of relevant intentions. This view is shared by Skinner et al. (1984) who designed the *Edinburgh Functional Communication Profile* (EFCP) in an attempt to structure observation and analysis of the communication strategies used by aphasic individuals making specific reference to context, modality and degree of success.

For speech and language therapists, one of the primary concerns has always been to improve communicative effectiveness of the individual's treatment. In attempting to meet this goal, the intervention strategies used must continually bear this concern in mind to ensure that remediation goals are mutually acceptable to both the client and society. However, until recently, much of this societal perspective was lost, perhaps in the name of objectivity and accountability. Prutting and Kirchner (1983), among others, have pointed out the need to view communication disorders from a social perspective, taking context into account rather than attempting to control it.

A note of caution has been sounded by Penn (1983) who warns that, since the social context of communication is so redundant, we may be overestimating the ability of the aphasic person. Communicative competence compared to linguistic competence may thus best be viewed as less impaired in aphasia rather than supposing that it remains intact. The most comprehensive linguistic study based on pragmatic theory appears to be that by Penn (1983) who developed a *Profile of Communicative Appropriateness* (PCA) based upon a comprehensive taxonomy derived from child language literature. Penn (1985) describes the PCA as 'a linguistic profile designed to characterize the communicative competence of a clinical subject' (p. 19). It was developed to identify the features of communication evading description by traditional methods. It is concerned primarily with language use beyond the sentence level and is based on a number of theoretical assumptions from the field of pragmatics, including the communicative context, conversational maxims (such as quality, quantity, relevance and manner) and the rules of communication. Penn (1985) argues that although there has been a reluctance on the part of linguistics to incorporate such contextual factors into a model of language, there is ample evidence to suggest that many aspects of communicative competence are amenable to analysis and can be systematically described and related. A major concept underlying the PCA is the notion of appropriateness. The language behaviour of an individual may only be judged as being appropriate within the context of the communicative event. The term 'appropriate' implies a societal framework of judgement based on the performance of the individual in a social context, rather than on his ability on all or none of the measures of language by items in a traditional test. In the opinion of Penn (1985) the perceived impact of an aphasic person's difficulty cannot be evaluated in terms of a score or a quantitative measure, but in terms of qualitative appropriateness. Penn's data (1983), suggest that there is relative independence of the syntactic and pragmatic aspects of aphasia. This finding, according to Goldblum (1985) raises two important issues: first, it casts some doubt on the validity of traditional classification schemes and their ability to reflect communicative competence, and, second, it highlights the need to consider structural and functional data together to facilitate a more comprehensive evaluation of the communicative competence of an aphasic person.

In a further contrast to previous measures, the *Pragmatic Protocol*, (Prutting 1982) examines the individual's pragmatic strengths and deficits within conversational discourse, and across a variety of contexts. The *Speech Act Theory* of Searle (1969) constitutes the framework underlying this *Pragmatic Protocol* which looks at behaviours under the categories of the utterance act, the propositional act and the illocutionary and perlocutionary acts. Since the *Pragmatic Protocol* is a societal appraisal rather than a clinical appraisal, the judgement is made as to whether the behaviour is penalising. The investigator must decide whether society will penalise an individual for exhibiting a particular behaviour. Thus, a behaviour may be incorrect but not necessarily judged as inappropriate (Prutting and Kirschner, 1983). A similar rating judgement was used in the EFCP (Skinner et al., 1984) to obtain an estimate of an individual's adequacy of communicative effectiveness.

An example of the potential for future development: the REFCP*

The REFCP incorporates the theoretical changes made to the EFCP (Skinner et al., 1984) as a result of its clinical use over a period of four years and incorporates formal suggestions and feedback from collaborating therapists in the USA and UK and informal feedback from other users. The contexts for the EFCP were initially developed from study of Halliday's (1975) functions of language with adaptations from Coggins and Carpenter's (1978) definition of pragmatic categories in pre-verbal and non-verbal children. Halliday's model divides language into seven categories: instrumental, regulatory, personal, interactional, heuristic, imaginative and representational. The authors hypothesised that, in the clinic, aphasic people restrict their usage to the 'instrumental' and 'personal' functions of language whilst demonstrating that in other situations they are able to use language for 'interactional' purposes. Like the *Pragmatic Protocol* of Prutting, the REFCP is based on speech act theory where there are two elements: the proposition and the illocutionary force. Both these elements are included in the interaction analysis section which is designed for individuals who have severely disrupted interactional patterns and who may use multiple modalities to communicate.

An underlying criticism of all functional assessments is that of subjectivity. The authors of the REFCP have attempted to answer this criticism by including the opportunity to collect quantitative data as well as qualitative information, through the interaction analysis section. The interaction analysis allows the clinician to score performance according to very basic criteria by measuring an observable feature — the

*(Wirz, Skinner and Dean, 1990).

effectiveness of the aphasic person's contribution in maintaining the interaction. The analysis categorises responses by type of speech act and modality of response. This kind of information can be used to document change over time or for comparison across individuals. When completing such an analysis, 10 conversational exchanges are required to be scored. A conversational exchange is defined as a contribution by one participant followed by a contribution from the other participant, including silence. The individual's contribution to each exchange is scored on a scale from 0–5, where 0 is communication breakdown and 5 is elaborate extension of the interaction.

During the design and trials of the REFCP, in order to verify that 10 conversational exchanges were sufficient to obtain a representative sample of communicative behaviour, at least 16 minutes of conversation were videotaped for each six aphasic individuals. Every interaction that occurred during these samples was coded and then individually rated by the authors. Each author rated a different set of 10 exchanges and the modal rating of each conversational sample was obtained. Analysis of the data revealed a high correlation between the modal figures for the complete conversational samples and each set of 10 conversational exchanges. Following this it was decided to use the strategy of rating 10 conversational exchanges in REFCP protocol. This was quicker and easier than a longer sample and gave very similar information.

A second profile possible from the REFCP is the communicative performance analysis which, in contrast to the interaction analysis, is based on a free conversation sample rather than 10 conversational exchanges. There is no restriction on the length or content of the sample. The individual's communicative behaviour is evaluated on three dimensions concerned with:

- Use of certain communicative functions.
- Effectiveness of communication.
- The modalities used to communicate.

The purpose is to record evidence of communicative potential — evidence that may be obtained in several different contexts over a period of time.

The emphasis on multi-modality communication is another area in which the REFCP differs from other published profiles. The modalities assessed are: speech, gesture, facial expression, vocalisation and writing, including drawing and symbol systems. These are considered the modalities most likely to be used spontaneously to circumvent communication difficulties and they are also the modalities most frequently employed in alternative and augmentative communication systems. Many communicators employ more than one modality to communicate and it has been found useful to observe whether communicative effectiveness is improved when two or more modalities are combined in an attempt to convey a message. The REFCP allows several modalities to be profiled, enabling the clinician to compare the effectiveness of different individual modalities available to the aphasic person and to analyse the combined effect of several modalities.

In some instances, especially when assessing severely impaired communicators, it has proved difficult to collect a sample of sufficient size. In an attempt to overcome this problem the REFCP includes the supplementary interview which provides structured scenarios used to elicit communicative functions not observed in spontaneous conversation. These scenarios, or prompts, allow the assessor to elicit the communicative functions in structured contexts if the REFCP is being re-administered periodically to document progress.

The REFCP also includes opportunities to profile the client's ability to repair an utterance. The authors believe that much of the success of communicative interaction with communicatively impaired individuals depends on how well the client attempts to revise responses that are inadequate or misunderstood by the listener. From a therapeutic point of view, it is important to know how such individuals cope in situations where they need to convey a request clearly, are asked for clarification or require clarification of something said to them. Wirz et al. (1989, 1990) believe that it is necessary to analyse the ability of a client to repair misunderstood messages and to document what changes are made to the original message following a query.

Very little has been written about the ability of the aphasic individual to use repair strategies but in the literature on child language disorders, Howell and Dean (1991), in particular, stress their importance in developing metalinguistic awareness in children with phonological impairment. They define repair as being the process by which we review, revise and correct our utterances to facilitate understanding.

The ability to repair language has been observed in normally developing children from about 18 months of age and Clark and Andersen (1979) provide evidence of self-monitoring and repair collected from the spontaneous conversations of 2- and 3-year-old children. Phonological repairs are reported as being the first to occur but decrease as children get older and are replaced in turn with morphological, lexical and, finally, syntactical repairs. Iwamura (1980) provides data to show that children will comment on and correct what other children say, demonstrating their awareness of the correctness or otherwise of certain linguistic forms. It has been noted in clinical experience that some aphasic individuals do not seem to use this strategy of repair spontaneously but can be taught to do so as part of a remediation programme. The authors of the REFCP believe it is important that such information is recorded as a component of communicative effectiveness.

The above studies highlight the many different communicative competences which can be profiled and give evidence of the value of such assessments when used by skilled clinicians. They point to a need to consider and define the range of pragmatic aspects of language in relation to other aspects of language (see Foldi, Cicone and Gardner, 1983; Prutting and Kirchner, 1983). More all-encompassing and dynamic intervention goals could emerge from such studies which would aim to enhance structural and functional aspects of communication in relationship to one another. Since competence lies within this relationship, the dyad is necessarily the unit of analysis where behaviours are judged in terms of societal appropriateness rather than clinical criteria of correctness. As these criteria take note of the environmental and cultural values surrounding the aphasic person, the speech and language therapist's criteria for discharge from intervention will need to be considered so that discharge occurs when the client can manage his relationships in a personally appropriate and effective manner, within the limitations imposed by his language impairment. Furthermore, intervention goals can emerge directly from the results of the profiles outlined above. The use of these tools serves to highlight the residual compensatory strengths of each individual, rather than concentrating on his inaccuracies and linguistic limitations and lead to intervention goals which are based on strengths rather than deficits.

References

Aten, J., Caligiuri, M. and Holland, A. (1982) The efficacy of functional communication therapy for chronic aphasia patients. *Journal of Speech and Hearing Disorders*, 47, 93–96

Bate, C. (1982) The pragmatics of language. *Communication Disorders*, VII, 2, 17–30

Behrman, M. and Penn, C. (1984) Non-verbal communication of aphasic patients. *British Journal of Disorders of Communication*, 19, 155–168

Brumfitt, S. and Clarke, P. (1983) An application of psychotherapeutic techniques to the management of aphasia. In: Code, C. and Muller, D. (eds). *Aphasia Therapy*, London: Edward Arnold

Clark, E.V. and Anderson, E.S. (1979) Spontaneous repairs: awareness in the process of acquiring language. *Child Language Development*, 16, 1–12

Coelho, C.A. and Duffy, R.J. (1987) The relationship of the acquisition of manual signs to severity of aphasia: a training study. *Brain and Language*, 31, 328–345

Coggins, T. and Carpenter, R. (1978) Categories for coding pre-speech intention communication. Unpublished manuscript. Seattle: University of Washington

Davis, G. (1989) Pragmatics and cognition in the treatment of language disorders. In: Seron, X. and Deloche, G. (eds). *Cognitive Approaches in Neuropsychological Rehabilitation*. Hillsdale, NJ: LEA

Davis, G. and Wilcox, M. (1981) Incorporating parameters of natural conversation in aphasia treatment. In: Chapey, R. (Ed.). *Language Intervention Strategies in Adult Aphasia*. (1st edition), Baltimore: Williams & Wilkins

Davis, G. and Wilcox, M. (1985) *Adult Aphasia Rehabilitation: Applied Pragmatics*. Windsor: NFER-Nelson

Dean, E.C., Skinner, C.M. and Edmonstone, A. (1987) An efficacy study of functional communication therapy: preliminary findings. *Proceedings of the First European Conference on Aphasiology*. Vienna, Austria

Duffy, R.J. and Liles, B.Z. (1979) A translation of Finkelberg's (1870) lecture on aphasia as 'asymbolia' with commentary. *Journal of Speech and Hearing Disorders*, 44 156–168

Edelman, G. (1983) PACE. *Bulletin: College of Speech Therapists*, **380**, 1–3

Ferro, J.M., Mariano, M.G., Castro-Caldas, A. and Santos, M.E. (1980) Gesture recognition in aphasia: a recovery study. *Journal of Clinical Neuropsychology*, **2**, 277–292

Feyereisen, F. and Seron, X. (1982a) Nonverbal communication and aphasia: a review. I Comprehension. *Brain and Language*, **16**, 191–212

Feyereisen, F. and Seron, X. (1982b) Nonverbal communication and aphasia: a review. II Expression. *Brain and Language*. **16**, 213–236

Foldi, N.S., Cicone, M. and Gardner, H. (1983) Pragmatic aspects of communication in brain-damaged patients. In: Segalowitz, S.J. (Ed.). *Language Functions and Brain Organization*. New York: Academic Press

Goldblum, G.M. (1985) Aphasia: a societal and clinical appraisal of pragmatic and linguistic behaviours. *South African Journal of Communication Disorders*, **32**, 11–18

Gravel, J. and LaPoint, L. (1982) Rate of speech of health-care providers during interactions with aphasic and non-aphasic individuals. In: Brookshire, R. (Ed.). *Clinical Aphrasiology Conference Proceedings*. Minneapolis: BRK

Green, G. (1982) Assessment and treatment of the adult with severe aphasia: aiming for functional generalisation. *Australian Journal of Communication Disorders*, **10**, 11–23

Green, G. (1984) Communication in aphasia therapy: some of the procedures and issues involved. *British Journal of Disorders of Communication*, **19**, 35–46

Grunwell, P. (1981) *The Nature of Phonological Disability in Children*. New York: Academic Press

Gurland, G., Chwat, S. and Wollner, S. (1982) Establishing a communication profile in adult aphasia: analysis of communicative acts and conversational sequences. In: Brookshire, R. (Ed.). *Clinical Aphasiology Conference Proceedings*. Minneapolis: BRK

Halliday, M.A.K. (1975) *Learning How to Mean: Explorations in the Development of Language*. New York: Elsevier North Holland

Helm-Estabrooks, N.A., Fitzpatrick, P.M. and Barresti, B. (1981) Visual action therapy for global aphasia. *Journal of Speech and Hearing Disorders*, **47**, 385–389

Herrman, M., Reichle, T., Lucins-Hoene, G., Wallesch, C.W. and Johannsen-Horbach, H. (1988) Non-verbal communication as a compensative strategy for severely nonfluent aphasics? — a quantitive approach. *Brain and Language*, **33**, 41–54

Herrman, M., Koch, U., Johannsen-Horbach, H. and Wallesch, C-W. (1989) Communicative skills in chronic and severe non-fluent aphasia. *Brain and Language*, **37**, 339–352

Holland, A. (1977) Some practical considerations in aphasia therapy. In: Sullivan, M. and Holland, A. (1982) Observing functional communication of aphasic adults. *Journal of Speech and Hearing Disorders*, **47**, 50–56

Howell, J. and Dean, E. (1991). *Treating Phonological Disorders in Children: Metaphon — Theory to Practice*. London: Whurr Publishers

Iwamura, O. (1980) *The Verbal Games of Pre-School Children*. London: Croom Helm

Karilahti, M. (1987) The effects of context on aphasics' expressive communication strategies. *Proceedings of the First European Conference on Aphasiology*. Vienna, Austria

Le May, A., David, R. and Thomas, A.P. (1988) The use of spontaneous gesture by aphasic patients. *Aphasiology*, 2, 2, 137–145

Lesser, R. and Milroy L. (1987) Two frontiers in aphasia therapy. *Bulletin of the College of Speech Therapists*, 420, 1–4

Parsons, C., Lambier, J., Snow, P., Couch, D. and Mooney, L. (1989) Conversational skills in closed head injury. Part I. *Australian Journal of Human Communication Disorders*, 17, 2, 37–46

Penn, A.C. (1983) Syntactic and pragmatic aspects of aphasic language. Unpublished doctoral dissertation. University of Witwatersvand

Penn, C. (1985) The profile of communicative appropriateness: a clinical tool for the assessment of pragmatics. *South African Journal of Communication Disorders*, 32, 18–32

Penn, C. (1988) The profiling of syntax and pragmatics in aphasia. *Clinical Linguistics and Phonetics*, 2, 179–207

Prinz, P. (1980) A note on requesting strategies in adult aphasics. *Journal of Communication Disorders*, 13, 65–73

Prutting, C. (1982) Pragmatics as social competence. *Journal of Speech and Hearing Disorders*, 47, 123–134

Prutting, C.A. and Kirchner, D.M. (1983) Applied pragmatics. In: Gallagher, T.M. and Prutting, C.A. (eds). *Pragmatic Assessment and Intervention Issues in Language*, San Diego, CA: College Hill Press

Prutting, C.A. and Kirchner, D. (1987) A clinical appraisal of the pragmatic aspects of language. *Journal of Speech and Hearing Disorders*, 52, 105–119

Sarno, M.T. (1969) *The Functional Communication Profile: New York Institute of Rehabilitative Medicine*. New York: University Medical Center

Schlanger, P. and Freimann, R. (1979) Pantomime therapy with aphasics. *Aphasia Apraxia Agnosia*, 1, 2, 34–39

Searle, J. (1969) *Speech Acts: An Essay in the Philosophy of Language*. Cambridge: Cambridge University Press

Simmons, N. (1986) Beyond standardised measures: special tests, language in context and discourse analysis in aphasia. *Seminars in Speech and Language*, 7, 181–205

Skelly, M. (1979) *Amerind Gestural Code based on Universal American Indian Hand Talk*, New York: Elsevier North Holland

Skinner, C., Wirz, S., Thomson, I. and Davidson, J. (1984) *The Edinburgh Functional Communication Profile: An Observation Procedure for the Evaluation of Disordered Communication in Elderly Patients*. Winslow: Winslow Press

Wilcox, M.J. and Davis, G.A. (1977) Speech act analysis of aphasic communication in individual and group settings. In: Brookshire, R.H. (Ed.). *Clinical Aphasiology Conference Proceedings*. Minneapolis: BRK

Wirz, S., Dean, E.C. and Benham, F. (1989) Towards an understanding of communicative effectiveness in aphasia. Institute of Neurology Research Report LOCR No. 1022. London: University of London

Wirz, S., Skinner, C.M. and Dean, E.C. (1990) *The Revised Edinburgh Functional Communication Profile*. Tucson: Communication Skill Builders

Chapter 6
The interactive skills of young communication aid users

Sandy Winyard

When clients use communication aids to supplement or augment their communication it is vital that the speech and language therapist should take the widest possible view of communicative strengths and needs. The therapist uses perceptual skills to observe her client's communicative attempts, communicative needs, communicative failings and difficulties and, in addition, to discover the communicative needs and frustrations of carers as well as the settings in which the client lives.

It was originally thought that introducing a communication aid to a non-verbal physically disabled child would be like providing a short-sighted child with glasses or a hearing impaired child with a hearing aid. At first, it seemed surprising that such children did not start to communicate easily now they had the means to do so. When examined more closely, however, it became obvious that communicating with a communication aid was a very complex process which and depended on many factors. For example, an accurate multi-disciplinary assessment was needed to recommend the communication aid that was best suited to the needs and skills of the child (Jones et al., 1990). Moreover, the successful introduction of a communication aid depended not only on a good multi-disciplinary assessment but also on the ability of the child's carers to support and encourage him and his system in his environment (Harris, 1982; Calculator, 1988; Light, 1989; Lombardino and Langley, 1989). This example explains why the high expectations of early communication aids have not been realised.

Successful use of a communication aid depends on a matrix of factors concerning the child, the aid or aids available to him, the methods he employs to use or access the communication aid, and the expectations, attitudes and support offered in his home and school environment.

The children discussed in this chapter are likely to use a symbol system and/or an electronic communication aid. They are generally too physically disabled to sign, although they may make use of some gross gesturing. They may vocalise and use some recognisable, meaningful vocalisations, but essentially they are non-verbal. Their main communicative need is seen as a lack of expressive ability. The communication aids selected for such children should fill this need and become their main expressive mode, or be part of a multi-modal system.

Communication aids fall into a number of categories:

1. Signing systems which are only useful if the child has the physical control to be able to sign fairly accurately.
2. Symbol systems which are particularly useful for more physically handicapped children.
3. Electronic aids which are useful for any child who has difficulties with verbal expression. These range from very simple devices to complex text-to-speech aids which, potentially, offer infinite expressive ability.

Most communication aid users need more than one communication aid, e.g. a visual display or synthetic speech system for spontaneous communication and a form of written output for schoolwork. A number of children combine gestures or simple signs, vocalisations, symbol systems and an electronic communication aid.

An important aspect of the communication aid is making it work for the individual user. Methods of accessing communication aids can be divided into two main categories — direct and indirect:

1. *Direct access*—the child selects the item for communication in one or, if the child is using a coded system, sometimes more movements. Examples of direct access would be fist-, finger- or eye-pointing or use of a head or light pointer for a symbol board. A traditional keyboard could be operated with fingers or a head pointer, or a non-traditional keyboard, such as a concept keyboard, could be operated with the fists.
2. *Indirect access*—the child has to use some method of scanning. This access is usually necessary when the child has very poor physical control and coordination. Examples of scanning methods could be using another person to scan down a symbol chart, stopping him on the correct horizontal line then scanning across and stopping him when the appropriate picture, symbol, word or letter is reached. Scanning can be done by use of a switch to stop the scanning process vertically and horizontally. There are a number of computer programmes which will do this, from simple games and puzzles to sophisticated wordprocessing programmes.

Any form of direct access is much quicker for the child and gives him a much greater degree of independence. Indirect access is slow and frequently relies on help from a carer. Clearly, selection of the best access system for the child is very important as, if the communication aid is not easy to use, clinical experience and natural observation strongly suggest that it will not be used.

There have been few follow-up studies on the outcome of the prescription of communication aids. Those that have been reported tend to support clinical observations from therapists and reports from schools and parents, that communication aids frequently do not meet client expectations and needs. Kraat (1985) compiled data on communicative interaction between communication aid users and natural speakers. She identified consistent trends, including limited use of communication aids and a reduced range of communicative functions, in users. Culp et al. (1986) carried out a retrospective survey of clients who had attended an augmentative communication aid service. Data showed that there was a low percentage of use of communication aids and a high percentage of their rejection. In addition, it was noted that children were much more likely to use a communication aid at school than at home. Udwin and Yule (1990; 1991a; 1991b) studied two groups of children learning to communicate using either Bliss symbols or Makaton signing, and followed them for 18 months. They report a disappointing picture of limited communication skills, with very little progress over time. They also comment on the very limited training practices in schools.

Such studies beg the question, 'Why don't these children communicate effectively with their aid?'.

The first point of possible breakdown is in the assessment and recommendation of the communication aid itself. Is the communication aid the right one for the child's needs? There have been a number of attempts to develop models for assessing this client group for the right communication aid. For example, Shane and Bashir (1980) offer an election decision matrix with 10 categories, including motor, language, cognitive and environmental factors. This matrix gives a decision to elect, reject or delay implementation of an augmentative communication system decision. In 1983, Ferrier and Shane extended this model to select a system for the client. The selection model takes account of environmental, user and technique factors.

It is vital that therapists consider all aspects of assessment, not just the child. One model, used by this author when considering the interactive skills of young communication aid users, is described in detail by Jones et al. (1990). It was developed by the Communication Aids Centre Team at The Wolfson Centre, London. The model recommends use of a pre-assessment questionnaire which examines the areas of visual attention and function, verbal comprehension, cause and effect, and communicative intent. If a child is seen to have the prerequisites, he is offered an assessment appointment. A first assessment usually takes a day. In the morning the child and his carers are seen by a multi-disciplinary team, consisting of an occupational therapist, a paediatrician, a psychologist, a rehabilitation engineer, and a speech and language therapist. In the afternoon the child's local therapists and teachers are invited to join the family. Before the child is seen, the family and the team meet to discuss him, how the family perceive his problems and how they feel he can best be helped.

Assessment by the multi-disciplinary team

A full assessment considers a number of areas, including:

1. Mobility — if the child is wheelchair-bound, the communication aid could be mounted on his wheelchair. If the child is mobile, the aid must be portable.
2. Posture — position is very important for accessing the communication aid.
3. Access — if the child has good hand function, he will be able to access a keyboard directly to work his communication aid. If the child has limited hand function, he could access his communication aid indirectly by use of switches. If the child does not have reliable hand function, the team need to identify another reliable, consistent response which may be trained.
4. Vision — it is important to know about the child's visual field because of positioning the communication aid's visual display. Many of the children referred have restricted visual fields.
5. Oculo-motor — the child's ability to scan needs to be assessed to ensure the size and type of visual display chosen is suitable.
6. Hearing — if the child has a hearing impairment it may be important to reinforce his auditory input with a visual means of communication, such as signing or use of symbols.
7. Symbolic and verbal comprehension — the child's comprehension level is assessed informally by use of developmental levels and formally by use of tests that do not require a verbal reply, such as the *Test for the Reception of Grammar* (TROG) (Bishop, 1983) and the *British Picture Vocabulary Scale* (BPVS) (Dunn, Pantile and Whetton, 1982).
8. Communicative functions — the range and type of communicative functions used.
9. Communicative modes — the modes and combination of modes the child uses for communicating, e.g. verbal, vocal, gestures, signs, symbols.

At the end of the day at The Wolfson Centre, the assessment team makes recommendations for a communication system that will meet the needs of the child and his environment.

Harris (1982) highlighted the difficulties that face communication aid users. She identified a minimum of eight steps the user has to take to express an idea, in contrast with three for a non-aid user. The vocal communicator can move from thought/idea to cognitive formulation and thus to the vocal expression of a thought/idea, whereas the communication aid user has to select which mode of expression he will use, alert the receiver as to the mode chosen, select the appropriate vocabulary and the appropriate sequencing of the message and, finally, check the accuracy of his choices *before* expressing himself. Figures 6.1 and 6.2 contrast the communicative planning of the vocal communicator with the much longer planning process of a non-vocal communicator.

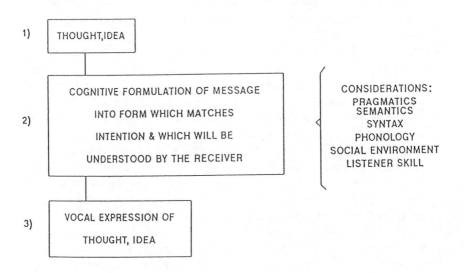

Figure 6.1 Intention to expression for vocal communicators (after Harris, 1982).

Harris (1982) also notes a number of potential barriers to effective interaction for the communication aid user that would fall into the categories of communication skills mentioned above and acceptance in his environment. Speed of communication is one — communication aid users are much slower than normal speakers. This can make the interaction boring and tedious and tempts the vocal partner to speak for the user. The listener–speaker roles get confused as, unless a speech synthesiser is being used, the vocal partner will need to speak the words and assemble the message that the communication aid user is indicating. This means that traditional turntaking is upset. Equality of interaction is lost and there is control by the vocal partner, who can anticipate, change the subject and dominate the interaction. Harris (1982) also comments that communication aids themselves are considerable barriers to effective communication because they are so unnatural, and both the user and the communicative partner need a working knowledge and an adequate level of skill to be able to use them.

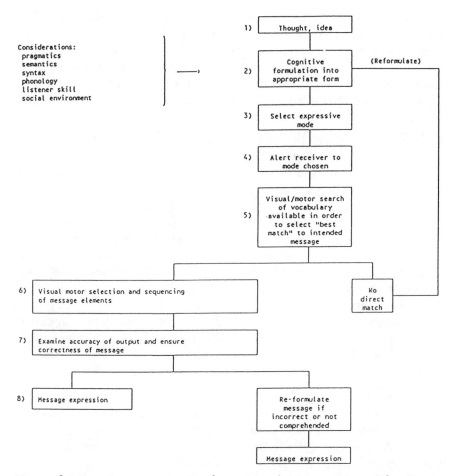

Figure 6.2 Intention to expression for non-vocal communicators (after Harris, 1982).

Evaluation of communication aid intervention: the Wolfson Centre Communication Aid Centre project

To evaluate how the child uses his communication aid it is necessary to observe the child in his natural environment. A follow-up study of nine children was initiated by the author. For children, two important environments are school and the home and it was decided to observe and record by videotape the child interacting with a teacher and a parent. It was important to know not only how the child was using his communication aid but also whether his communication had changed since its introduction. Recordings were therefore taken at the time of assessment (before recommendations for a communication system had been made) and approximately one year later when it was expected that the recommendations would have been implemented.

The resulting video recordings were analysed by use of a descriptive profile of communication patterns that was developed at the Wolfson Centre for this client group (Allen, 1988; Winyard, 1993). The adult–child interaction was divided into communication acts and coding focused on:

1. Structure of interaction: each communication act in the discourse was coded as being an initiation or a response.
2. Communication rate: this was measured by calculating the number of communication acts that took place per minute.
3. Communicative functions: only the child's responses were coded for function. Functions were: social conventions; request for object or action; request for information; request for clarification; request for attention; confirmations and denials; provision of information; provision of clarification; expression of self; elicited imitation; turn-taking in a game; unintelligible (adapted from Light, Collier and Parnes, 1985).
4. Communicative mode: only the child's communication was coded for eight possible modes. Modes were: verbal, yes/no only; verbal, more than yes/no; vocal; gesture; sign; symbol; electronic aid; or physical.

Results of the analysis of this observation indicated that there were two main areas of concern. The first was with the child's communication skills, interaction and communicative function. The second with the unwillingness of people in the child's environment to accept and encourage the use of the communication aid.

Interestingly, it was felt by all parents and all but one teacher that the children had been provided with a communication aid that could meet their needs. This view was supported by the Communication Aids Centre team when they saw children for review. The children could use the aid, i.e. they could operate it and it was usually physically with them. However, seeing the child in his own environment (school and home) demonstrated very clearly that, although it was possible to communicate by use of the aid, the reality was either that it was not used or was used in a very limited way.

Communication skills

During the last 20 years there has been considerable interest and work in the area of pre-linguistic development. The importance of the non-verbal structural framework — early gestures and vocalisations — has been highlighted (Bruner, 1975; Bates, Camaioni and Volterra, 1975), as has the type of language input available to the child. (Snow, 1972; Nelson, 1973). Clarke-Stewart and Hevey (1981) studied social interaction in children aged 12–30 months and found that the child's communication increased during that time, whereas the mother's attention and communication first increased and then decreased as her child's communication increased. There has been tremendous growth in the number of studies involving normal children and their care-givers, but there still remains a dearth of studies which involve physically disabled children and their care-givers.

The work that has been done, however, suggests that there are differences in the interaction patterns between normal children and their care-givers and physically disabled children and their care-givers. Kogan and Tyler (1973) studied mother–child interaction in three groups of children: physically disabled; normal, and those with learning difficulties. They found that the mothers of the disabled children displayed more controlling behaviours than the mothers of the non-disabled children and that both groups of disabled children were more passive than the normal control group, although the physically disabled group displayed more assertive, controlling behaviour than the group with learning difficulties. In 1987, Barrera and Vella compared non-disabled and physically disabled infants and their mothers and found that physically disabled infants engaged in less eye contact than normal infants. They also noted, as did the previous studies of Kogan and Tyler (1973); Kogan, Tyler and Turner (1974) and Kogan (1980), that mothers of disabled infants were more controlling in their interaction with their children.

As the non-verbal framework has assumed such an important place in the development of communication it would seem that these differences in interaction patterns, which occur between physically disabled and non-physically disabled infants are of significance to the normal development of communication in this client group.

Certainly the observational data from the communication aids follow-up study (Winyard, 1993) and data from Udwin and Yule (1990; 1991a; 1991b) report that the children concerned are essentially passive communicators and language input is controlling and limited. This suggests that the interaction patterns displayed early in development are continued as the child grows older.

Results of the observation in schools and homes

The descriptive pattern of communication patterns used (Allen, 1988; Winyard, 1993), categorises the observed communication into: structure; rate of interaction; communicative functions and modes of communication.

Structure

At assessment the pattern of initiation and response was similar in both the parent–child and the teacher–child dyads. Parents and teachers produced approximately the same number of communication acts that fell into the initiations category as fell into the response category. Of the communication acts which children produced when interacting with both teachers and parents, a very small proportion were classified as initiations and a large proportion as responses. The follow-up picture was similar, although a slight increase in the number of child initiations is noted, in particular within the teacher–child dyad.

Table 6.1 Structure of the parent–child, teacher–child dyads*

Dyad	Adult initiation		Adult response		Child initiation		Child response	
	A	FU	A	FU	A	FU	A	FU
Parent–child	27.2	30.3	27.9	24.4	1.7	2.8	43.2	42.5
Teacher–child	28.9	30.3	28.3	26.1	2.0	5.2	40.8	38.4

*Mean (%) of total number of communication acts observed.
A = assessment; FU = follow-up.

Rate of interaction

At assessment and follow-up, the rate of interaction was similar, ranging between 19.4–22.2 communication acts/min. Foulds (1980) comments that a typical adult speaks at a rate of 126–172 words/min. The communication act as defined here can be more than one word or one non-verbal response, and the rate includes both communicative partners. However, in practice many of the acts were single words or vocalisations and, allowing for half the dyad speaking normally, the rate must be seen as very slow when compared to normal communicators. The teacher–child dyad produced a slightly slower mean than the parent–child dyad. This was probably due to the more formal setting of school when compared to home. Teachers displayed a greater inclination to wait for the child to communicate and were less keen to speak for him in the structured setting of the classroom.

Table 6.2 Rate of interaction: mean number of communication acts/min

Dyad	Time 1	Time 2
Parent–child	22.2	20.9
Teacher–child	21.6	19.4

Function

At assessment there was no difference in the children's use of functions when they were communicating with a parent or a teacher. Nearly 50% of the children's communicative functions fell into the category of confirmations and denials. Approximately one-third of the total functions recorded were coded as provision of information by answering a question which only has a few possible answers. A very small proportion of functions were coded as higher level functions. These higher level functions were: providing new information; clarifying misunderstandings; requesting information, and requesting clarification (cf. Dale, 1980; Light et al., 1985; Baumgart, Johnson and Helmstetter, 1990). There were so few instances of the remaining functions that they were collapsed into one category 'Other' for coding purposes. The follow-up picture was again very similar, with the exception of the category 'provision of information by answering a question that has a few possible answers' which showed a significant decrease in both parent–child and teacher–child dyads. This decrease was not reflected in a significant increase in the higher level functions, but in a spread of increase across all other function categories. This was felt to be a response to generally raising awareness about communication through the assessment and recommendation procedure.

Table 6.3 Use of function by the child in parent–child, teacher–child dyads*

Dyad	Confirmations denials		Answering questions (a) few possible —answers		Higher level functions		Other	
	A	FU	A	FU	A	FU	A	FU
Parent–child	46.2	51.7	34	24.2	5	7.2	14.8	16.9
Teacher–child	47	49.5	33	24.8	6.6	9.5	12.3	16.2

*Mean (%) of total number of functions observed.
A = assessment; FU = follow-up.

Modes of communication

Nine subjects completed the study and with the exception of one, who employed a multi-modal system, and two, who relied heavily on symbol systems, they demonstrated little consistent use of the communication systems available to them at assessment. They all had access to signing or symbol systems but preferred to communicate with very poor and largely unintelligible speech and vocalisations. At follow-up only two children had received a communication aid from health authority funding, and one of these was refusing to use it. One child had a communication aid on loan from the Communication Aids Centre and was using it to back up his unintelligible speech. The remaining six subjects' modes of communication were unchanged from the time of assessment.

Implications for the therapist at assessment

In summary, the children presented a communication pattern at assessment that was similar to the patterns displayed by the studies of physically disabled infants and their parents referred to above (Barrera and Vella, 1987; Kogan, 1980; Kogan and Tyler, 1973; Kogan, Tyler and Turner, 1974). They were passive communicators with a high proportion of responses to initiations, used a very restricted range of communicative functions and made limited use of any communication aid available to them. The study was intended to measure change in the children's communication after intervention with a communication aid, but delay in the provision of the recommended communication aid was a limiting factor. These delays are common and a national policy on regional loan banks is required to enable children to start using the communication aid they need immediately (Rowley et al., 1988)

Environment

Generally, at assessment the child's environment tended to emphasise the passivity of the child. Adults in the dyads were over-protective and controlling of the child's environment, tending to restrict communicative possibilities by asking many closed questions and frequently talking for the child. When the child did communicate he was often not encouraged to use the communication aid available.

Teachers made greater use of the communication aid but this tended to be at structured times, for particular activities. When visits to schools were made, children were often found with their communication chart/book in a bag on the back of their chair or their computer switched off or being used for another child. Parents often said they did not like the communication aid because they felt it made their child look more handicapped. One of the most frequent phrases used by parents about their child and his communication was 'we can understand him'. Even during the course of the assessment day this was often disproved, but it continued to be said. Teachers, parents and the child were usually looking for a high technology communication aid that would enable the child to 'talk'.

Responses to interview questions about the child's functional communication in everyday life revealed that teachers considered that the child used the communication aid more than the parent reported. Teachers also considered that the child could make himself understood to a wider range of people than the parent reported. This supports the observations of the Communication Aids Centre team that schools generally make more use of the communication aid than homes.

These observations led staff to consider that, in addition to assessment and recommendation of communication aids for the child, it would be beneficial to provide some training in communication skills for parents. Kogan (1980) had demonstrated that it was possible to change parental interactions with their children in a positive way, leading to a smaller number of stressful interactions and more behaviours that expressed warmth and acceptance.

Training

To the therapist it is clear that training of teachers and parents is vital. Allen (1988) used a case control study to evaluate the effects of a Workshop Training Day for parents. This aimed to inform parents about communication and make them more aware of their own communication, specifically when they were communicating with their child. It was hoped that the effects of the workshop would be seen through:

- Increased child initiations.
- Improved adult responses to child initiations.
- Extended range of communicative functions.
- Extended range of expressive modes.
- More frequent and consistent use of the communication system.
- Improved vocabulary.

The day began with an introduction to communication, using the Harris (1982) models of vocal and non-vocal communicators to demonstrate the huge difference in the expressive communication process between normal speakers and aided communicators. The main part of the morning was spent working in small groups using videotapes of parents and their children interacting. This method enabled parents to actually observe themselves communicating with their children. They were asked to:

- Identify two good points and three problem areas about communicating with their children.
- Think about practical ways of improving communication in those problem areas.
- Discuss with one of the speech and language therapists running the workshop, their observations and ideas and to begin to develop individual aims for each child.

In the afternoon there were opportunities for role play. These offered the chance to practise activities that facilitated good communication patterns. The final session of the day identified individual aims for each parent and child.

Allen (1988) followed up these children three months after the Workshop Training Day and Winyard (1993) followed up the groups approximately one year later. Short-term changes at 3 months were recorded. The training group showed improvements in all the target areas with the exception of an increase in initiations. Particularly noticeable at 3 months was a significant positive change in the appropriateness of adult responses to child initiations. This had decreased at the one-year follow-up but was still a considerable improvement on the baseline measure.

Table 6.4 Case control study: adult responses to child initiations*

Group	Time 1	Time 2	Time 3
Training	36.1	92.7	81.6
Control	51.6	65.6	54.5

*Mean (%) of possible child initiations.

It is clear from the above discussion that communication aids generally fall far short of expectations and often become another mode for the child to express his very limited communication. Many children just transfer the communicative patterns they are using to the new system. The people in their environment communicate with them in the same way and can often be heard to say 'Come on, use your aid' to communicate something like 'I want to go to the toilet' for which they have a perfectly understandable vocalisation.

Normal communicators use a number of communication modes. Although speech is usually their main mode, they also use gestures, facial expression and eye contact, write, and physically touch people and things. This is considered to be quite normal for vocal people, but is not as acceptable for non-vocal people who tend to be expected to communicate using only their most efficient (usually high technology) communication aid. The symbol board, few signs and vocalisations that used to be so useful are forgotten and not responded to in the rush to make the high technology communication aid work.

It is interesting to note that the one child who was progressing well in the follow-up study was using a multi-modal system. Both her parents and those in her home environment responded to her communication whether it was by vocalisation, signing or symbols. Her symbol chart was always available — beside her when she was engaged in an activity and she chose the mode to use to communicate. If she failed in one mode, she would often try again, supplementing her first mode with communication in another. This is normal. If a child's speech is not understood, he will try again with gestures or physically show you what he is talking about. Crucial to the successful working of this 'repair' function is the ability of the communicative partner to expect signals, e.g. if the vocal partner is only communicating via the communication aid, she will miss the eye-pointing that the child is doing. If the message is being misinterpreted, the eye-pointing might be the strategy that produces comprehension, in the same way that gesture might be the strategy that interprets the vocal child's speech.

Normal communication is active, dynamic and equal for both partners and this needs to be encouraged in both the communication aid user and those communicating with him. From reviewing the literature and observing physically disabled, non-verbal children as they develop, it can be seen that these components of interaction are at risk in this client group. Emphasis needs to be directed early in the assessment/ intervention process to balance the interaction between disabled infants and their care-givers, to encouraging equality and facilitating control in the child.

Communication risks should be taken by all communication partners of the child, in order to extend language competence and communicative function. This means limiting the questions which require a safe answer (provision of information, a few possible answers or a confirmation/denial). A conscious effort should be made to increase the communication input that requires the child to use higher-level functions, e.g. answering questions that require a new idea, requesting information, requesting clarification and repairing communication that has broken down. Studies show that communication aid users have a very restricted use of communicative functions. Udwin and Yule (1991a) reported that over 80% of all utterances recorded were for just four functions, and Winyard presents an even more depressing picture of approximately 80% of utterances with parents being for two functions. Neither of these studies demonstrated a relationship between language comprehension and poor expressive ability, indeed, they found that childrens' language comprehension was often within normal limits, but that expressive ability is limited by mode and use and acceptance of that mode.

For the vocal partner and the non-vocal partner to use the aid for communicating, both need to understand how it works and to be competent in its use. Understanding how a communication aid works involves more than switching it on or providing the symbol/word board. The content of the computer or symbol board has to meet the needs of the child and all the situations he will find himself in. Therefore, selecting the best vocabulary and, in the case of an electronic communication aid, programming it to predict words and structure is fundamental to its effective use. Allen et al. (1989) suggest many ideas for doing this.

We have already noted that speed is an important factor, and it may be that for communication aid users to become really effective they need to utilise some kind of shorthand or a predictive system, for example, good, fast Bliss board users usually communicate in a telegraphic way. Wordprocessing packages with predictive lexicons reduce the keystrokes users have to make and therefore reduce time. The *Predictive and Adaptive Lexicon* (PAL) (Swiffin, Arnott and Newell, 1988) is an example of this.

To use the system skill and practice are necessary, so are acceptance and adaptability. The vocal partner has to be alert for signals from all potential communication modes, but most importantly, the communication interaction must use the aids available and not bypass them. There is a great temptation to continue using the easy old system of asking the child '20 questions' to find out what he wants, to guess or talk for him, etc. This will severely limit his communication potential, both in function and communicative partners. If old patterns are continued his communication will only be understood by a very limited group of familiar people. He will never be able to communicate with people who do not know him well. One of the reasons for introducing a communication aid is to maximise opportunities for communication in all situations.

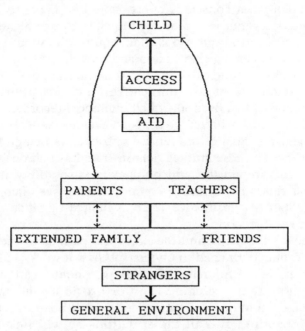

Figure 6.3 Possible expansions to patterns of communication. — old patterns; --- possible extensions to old patterns; ▬ new patterns with potential expansion.

When an electronic communication aid is provided for a child it is vital that intensive training is provided so that his communication is extended and developed, not restricted. (Calculator, 1988). In Winyard's (1993) follow-up study, the one child who had been provided with a communication aid by the health authority was using it and enjoying it. He had gained in independence as he could interact with strangers, but the quality of his interaction had decreased. At follow-up, his rate of interaction with his mother had decreased from 23 acts/min to 9 acts/min. This was because his access to the communication aid was through scanning which, certainly for the unskilled user, has an inverse relationship between speed and accuracy. Initiations and higher-level functions had decreased due to the predominant use of preprogrammed phrases which restrict the range and creativity of communication. Undoubtedly, lack of skill with the communication aid for both mother and child were factors here, as was a lack of professional help. An intensive training programme for the child, mother, and school about the system and its use could have made a huge impression on the introduction of this communication aid.

There is no doubt that using the system successfully for communication is very difficult. As Harris (1982) comments 'augmentative devices and techniques can pose barriers'. They are unnatural and generally do not facilitate spontaneous communication easily. Work is being carried out in this area as it is seen as fundamental to communication, e.g. *Conversation Helped by Automatic Talk* (CHAT) (Alm, Arnott and Newell, 1989; Newell, 1989). This system allows the user to access with one keystroke a suitable 'type' of remark, e.g. an acknowledgement. This kind of idea facilitates greater speed and more normal interaction. Perhaps one of the most useful interventions that can be made is to persuade speakers who interact with communication aid users that they must *wait* for the child to respond and give him time to make his communication aid work.

We are still a long way from the child's communication aid being seen in the same way as a pair of glasses, but this is the sort of relationship we should be aiming for. To encourage this we should be:

- Starting early.
- Using multi-modal systems.
- Building on the communication modes the child already uses.
- Expecting signals from all modes.
- Training interaction skills for both partners.
- Encouraging equality in turntaking.
- Extending and developing language functions.
- Facilitating the child's communication skills.
- Allowing the child control of the conversation.
- Taking communication risks.
- Providing knowledge about the communication aid.

- Practising the skills of using the communication aid.
- Giving the child time to communicate.

The communication aid is just another mode of expression. However, non-vocal children need a structured approach to learning to communicate with an aid. It is not as simple as being assessed, having a communication aid recommended, purchasing and using it. Even when the recommendations for equipment are right, using the aid for effective communication involves a complex matrix of skills and knowledge that both the child and those in his environment need to learn, practise and accept.

References

Allen, J.A. (1988) Teaching interaction skills to parents of aided communicators. Unpublished M.Sc. thesis. City University

Allen, J.A., Cockrill, H., Davies, E., Fuller, P., Jolleff, N., Larcher, J., Nelms, G. and Winyard, S. (1989) *Augmentative Communication: More than Just Words*. Oxford: Ace Centre Publications

Alm, N., Arnott, J.L. and Newell, A.F. (1989). Discourse analysis and pragmatics in the design of a conversation prosthesis. *Journal of Medical Engineering and Technology* 13, 10–12

Bates, E., Camaioni, L. and Volterra, V. (1975) The acquisition of performatives prior to speech. *Merrill-Palmer Quarterly* 21, 205–216

Barrera, M.E. and Vella, D.M. (1987) Disabled and non-disabled infants' interactions with their mothers. *American Journal of Occupational Therapy* 41, 168–172

Baumgart, D., Johnson, J. and Helmstetter, E. (1990) *Augmentative and Alternative Communication Systems for Persons with Moderate and Severe Disabilities*. Baltimore: Paul H. Brookes

Bishop, D. (1983) *Test for the Reception of Grammar*. Cambridge: MRC Applied Psychology Unit

Bruner, J. (1975) The otogenesis of speech acts. *Journal of Child Language* 2, 1–19

Calculator, S.N. (1988) Evaluating the effectiveness of AAC programs for persons with severe handicap. *Augmentative and Alternative Communication* 4, 177–179

Clarke-Stewart, K.A. and Hevey, C.M. (1981) Longitudinal relations in repeated observations of mother–child interaction from 1 to 2.5 years. *Developmental Psychology* 17, 127–145

Culp, D.M., Ambrosi, D.M., Berninger, T.M. and Mitchell, J.O. (1986) Augmentative communication aid use — a follow-up study. *Augmentative and Alternative Communication* 2, 19–24

Dale, P.S. (1980) 'Is early pragmatic development measurable?' *Journal of Child Language*, 7, 1–12

Dunn, L.M., Pantile, D. and Whetton, C. (1982) *British Picture Vocabulary Scale*. Windsor: NFER-Nelson

Ferrier, L.J. and Shane, H.C. (1983) A description of a non-speaking population under consideration for augmentative communication systems. In: Hogg, J. and Mittler, P.J. (eds). *Advances in Mental Handicap Research*, Vol. 2. London: John Wiley

Foulds, R.A. (1980) Communication rates for non-speech expression as a function of manual tasks and linguistic restraints. Proceedings of the International Conference on Rehabilitation Engineering, London

Harris, D. (1982) Communication interaction processes involving non-vocal physically handicapped children. *Topics in Language Disorders* 2, 21–37

Jones, S., Jolleff, N., McConachie, H. and Wisbeach, A. (1990) A model for assessment of children for augmentative communication systems. *Child Language Teaching and Therapy* 6, 305–321

Kogan, K.L. (1980) Intervention systems between preschool handicapped or developmentally delayed children and their parents. In: Field, T.M., Goldberg, S., Stern, D. and Sostek, A.M. (eds). *High Risk Infants and Children: Adult and Peer Interactions*. New York: Academic Press

Kogan, K.L. and Tyler, N. (1973) Mother–child interaction in young physically handicapped children. *American Journal of Mental Deficiency* 77, 492–497

Kogan, K.L., Tyler, N. and Turner, P. (1974) The process of interpersonal adaption between mothers and their cerebral palsied children. *Developmental Medicine and Child Neurology* 16, 518–527

Kraat, A. (1985) *Communication Interaction between Aid Users and Natural Speakers*. Lancing, MI: University Centre for International Rehabilitation

Light, J. (1989) Toward a definition of communicative competence for individuals using augmentative and alternative communication systems. *Augmentative and Alternative Communication* 5, 137–144

Light, J., Collier, B. and Parnes, P. (1985) Communicative interaction between young, non-speaking, physically disabled children and their primary caregivers. Part II: communicative function. *Augmentative and Alternative Communication* 1, 98–107

Lombardino, L. and Langley, M.B. (1989) Strategies for assessing severely multi-handicapped children for augmentative and alternative communication. *European Journal of Special Needs Education* 4, 157–170

Nelson, K. (1973) Structure and strategy in learning to talk. *Monographs of the Society in Research in Child Development* 38

Newell, A.F. (1989) PAL and CHAT, human interfaces for extraordinary situations. In: Salenieks, P. (Ed.). *Computing Technologies*. Hemel Hempstead: International Book Distributors

Rowley, C.M., Stowe, J., Bryant, J. and Chamberlain, M.A. (1988) Communication aid provision. *British Journal of Disorders of Communication* 23, 1–12

Shane, H.C. and Bashir, A.S. (1980) Election criteria for the adoption of an augmentative communication system: preliminary considerations. *Journal of Speech and Hearing Disorders* 45, 549–566

Snow, C. (1972) Mother's speech to children learning language. *Child Development* 43, 549–566

Swiffin, A.L., Arnott, J.L. and Newell, A.F. (1988) Adaptive and predictive techniques in a communication prothesis. *Augmentative and Alternative Communication* 3, 181–191

Udwin, O. and Yule, W. (1990) Augmentative communication systems taught to cerebral palsied children – a longitudinal study. I: The acquisition of signs and symbols, and syntactic aspects of their use over time. *British Journal of Disorders of Communication* 25, 295–310

Udwin, O. and Yule, W. (1991a) Augmentative communication systems to to cerebral palsied children – a longitudinal study. II: Pragmatic features of sign and symbol use. *British Journal of Disorders of Communication* 26, 137–148

Udwin, O. and Yule, W. (1991b) Augmentative communication systems taught to cerebral palsied children — a longitudinal study. III: Teaching practices and exposure to sign and symbol use in schools and homes. *British Journal of Disorders of Communication* 26, 149–162

Winyard, S. (1993) Communication patterns in non-verbal, physically disabled children — description and intervention. Unpublished M.Phil. dissertation. University of London

Chapter 7
Assessing the communication of clients with profound intellectual and multiple disabilities

Ann Edmonson

Introduction

It is tempting to think of people with profound intellectual and multiple physical disabilities as a homogeneous group who, because of their severe disabilities, function in a limited and similar manner, and are totally unable to communicate. Indeed, it is likely that they will have little or no speech. Leeming et al. (1978) found that one-third of children in ESN(S) schools in Manchester and Cheshire were at, or below, the level of imitating single words. Evans and Ware (1987), in a study of Special Care Units in the south-east of England, found that of the 800 children on whom information was available teachers reported 15.4% as using speech. However, care-givers and professionals who know such people have long recognised that, although they may have no speech, they are individuals each with their own personalities, likes and dislikes and range of emotions which they are able to communicate.

Through communication with people who have the skills to interact with them, people with profound intellectual and multiple physical disabilities are able to form relationships, but they are often misunderstood, misinterpreted and ignored by those who do not possess such skills. It is vital that the communication skills of people with profound intellectual and multiple physical disabilities are assessed effectively so that they can experience successful communication with a wider range of individuals and thus develop and extend the range of their communication.

Communication of clients with profound intellectual and multiple disabilities

It is evident that, as in mother–infant communication, if the profoundly handicapped person is to achieve successful communication, the competent communicator in the dyad must continuously monitor the individual's behaviours and interact in a sensitive, responsive manner. This behaviour is often intuitive in mother–infant communication with both normal and disabled children. However, the normal child is constantly developing, whereas the development of the person with severe learning difficulties is likely to be extremely slow or static. In order to facilitate and monitor development it is necessary to assess accurately all aspects of the client's communication and to analyse the strategies that the competent communicator in the dyad brings to the situation. Only by assessing both sides of the dyad carefully can therapy be directed towards developing the interaction skills of the client through intensive interaction therapy (Nind and Hewett, 1988; Watson and Knight, 1991; Knight, 1991). This chapter directs attention towards the assessment of both partners in the interaction.

The client with profound intellectual and multiple disabilities will function at a developmentally very young level, will often have limited movement and may also have additional sensory handicaps. Clients who are more physically able may also present with challenging behaviours, such as self-mutilation or aggression towards others. Where speech is present, it may be repetitive and inappropriate. Such clients have poorly developed interaction skills and, typically, their communication behaviour will consist of a small range of communication routines. Burford (1988) has described how, in spite of their disabilities, these people are able to communicate:

> Despite these impediments, people with profound mental handicaps are capable of participating and enjoying interactions with others as many investigators will attest. This basic emotional communication is similar to that observed between non-handicapped infants and their primary care givers (p. 189).

As Burford (1988) has identified, analogies can be drawn between the communication of profoundly multiply handicapped people and that of normal infants. Therefore the assessment and therapy for such individuals will be helped by a sound knowledge of research by developmental psychologists into infant–care-giver communication. Researchers, such as Trevarthon (1979) and Newson (1977), have demonstrated that the child is not the passive partner in the learning process as was previously thought. They argue that from birth the child is capable of complex organised behavioural sequences and that the pre-language skills learned in the first year of life form the foundation for communication in adult life. Newson (1979) describes how adult–child interactions are synchronised with each other, indicating that the child is biologically programmed to communicate. Trevarthon (1979) has described a stage in infant communication which he calls 'intersubjectivity', where the movements of the care-giver and child are coordinated and enable emotional communication. Burford (1988) argues that this style of communication is similar to that occurring between profoundly handicapped adults and their care-givers, and has identified 'action cycles', which she describes as 'rhythmic groups of cyclical movements', used by adults during interactions with profoundly handicapped children in order to involve and maintain interaction. These action cycles used by care-givers and infants have been found by Burford (1988) to be cross-cultural. Typically, profoundly handicapped individuals will present with a small range of communication routines or action cycles. Examples of such action cycles would include:

- Repetitive patting movements of the hands.
- Repetitive rubbing movements of the hands on the body.
- Head nodding.
- Rocking.

During mother–infant communication, the mother is particularly sensitive to the child's attention span and is able to hold and extend it by developing various communication strategies. Brazelton, Koslowski and Main (1974) entitled this the 'holding framework'. Schaffer (1977) has described how the mother sustains an interaction with her child:

> Early interactive sequences generally begin with the infant's own sponta-
> neous behaviour that the mother then chimes in to support, repeat, consent
> upon and elaborate his response ... she holds herself ready to let the infant
> resume as soon as he wishes (p. 294).

Schaffer (1977) has identified different strategies used by mothers which he calls: phasing, adaptive, facilitative, elaborative, initiating and control techniques. These techniques are used by mothers when interacting with their babies. Other strategies used by mothers include imitation (Pawlby, 1977), exaggeration, repetition and slowing down her actions (Stern, 1977). All these activities help to maintain the child's attention and enable the child to develop the joint-attention described by Bruner (1977) which is so important for further development. In addition, because the mother's responses to the child are contingent on his behaviour, they enable him to learn intentionally. Once intentionality is learned, which Bates, Camaioni and Volterra (1975) argue is connected with the awareness of means–end relationships, the way is paved for the development of pointing, gesture and the acquisition of first meanings and symbolic functioning.

Assessment

Speech and language therapists have assessed clients with profound learning difficulties for many years, using their skills and their knowledge of early communication development. Each therapist has devised her own particular method of doing this. Such assessments have often been undervalued, and criticised as being 'subjective', 'unscientific', and qualitative rather than quantative. There has been a trend towards the use of standard published assessment rather than recording the observations of behaviour in a less structured but possibly more comprehensive and client-specific way. King (1989) has described how pragmatic assessments tend to use one of three approaches:

1. Ethnographic approach — emphasises assessment of the child within a natural setting, with the assessor taking the role of observer (passive).
2. Checklists — look at verbal, non-verbal and paralinguistic aspects of communication.
3. Standardised tests (p. 192).

Most commercially available assessments for clients with profound intellectual and multiple disabilities tend to fall into the first two categories.

The *Affective Communication Assessment* (Coupe et al., 1987) could perhaps be included in the first category. This very useful assessment involves the client being presented with stimuli or experiences that are likely to elicit strong positive or negative responses. People who know the client will then interpret this response. A range of communicative behaviours are then identified and these behaviours can then be extended and developed through consistent responses to them.

The *Pre-verbal Communication Schedule* (Kiernan and Reid, 1987) is a checklist of communication behaviours to be carried out with the client's care-giver. After completion of the checklist, the therapist is then able to plot the results on a developmental chart, which allows analysis of skills involved in communication, or on a graph of communication functions.

The *Pragmatics Profile of Early Communication Skills* (Dewart and Summers, 1988) uses an interview format to elicit descriptive information about the client's communication skills under the headings:

- Communicative interactions.
- Responses to communication.
- Interaction and conversation.
- Contextual variation.

These assessments are all valuable tools for the speech and language therapist. None of the commercially available assessments, however, take account of the strategies used by the competent communicator in the dyad. The strategies of the competent communicator are essential to ensure successful communication with the individual with profound intellectual and multiple physical disabilities and should be analysed alongside those of the person with multiple disabilities. Communication is, after all, a two-way process. The assessment of these clients can be as complex as any linguistic assessment. These are clients who cannot be relied upon to respond in a consistent way to a particular task, therefore assessment is not simply a matter of presenting them with a task and noting their response. Rather profoundly disabled people can be better understood by *observing* their behaviour.

Murphy (1987) suggests that when using observation as an assessment tool in the functional analysis of people with learning difficulties it is important to consider what sort of observational techniques are being used. She suggests six different types of observation techniques. All may be appropriate at different times with the same client if the therapist is to build up a full picture of the client's communicative abilities.

The six types of observation suggested by Murphy (1987) are:

1. *Contributor's Methods*: requiring observers to watch and record during the observation period.
2. *Descriptive Recording*: the observer is interested in only one (or a few) behaviours and describes these.
3. *Event Recording*: the observer notes the occurrence of specific behaviour(s) which have been pre-determined as being of interest.
4. *Duration Recording*: events are timed either to produce a cumulative total or different events are timed and recorded separately.
5. *Sophisticated Continuous Methods*: using either elaborate recording equipment or indeed elaborate paper and pencil recording methods.
6. *Discontinuous Methods*: observation entailing repeated time sampling.

The methods of observation suggested in this chapter fall into Murphy's 'descriptive recording' category.

Detailed assessment information is accumulated over a matter of weeks, or even months, of observation. It should take place within an interactive framework, so that the process is meaningful for the client. The speech and language therapist must have built up a relationship with the client and his carers over a number of interactive sessions so that she has become familiar with the client's repertoire of communication behaviours. Such an assessment should attempt to describe the quality of an interactive exchange where both communicators are fully 'engaged' and when emotional communication is taking place. This involves describing qualitative aspects, such as body proximity, bodily tension or physical contact, as well as eye contact, facial expression and other parameters (described in more detail later in this chapter). Additionally, a full assessment should collate this information from all the competent communicators involved with the client so that a complete picture of his communicative abilities is built up.

Assessment method

The method proposed here has been devised through work with profoundly disabled clients in Edinburgh and consists of recording those strategies and action cycles identified by the competent communicator during interactive exchanges which contribute to successful communication with the client. This list of strategies should be updated constantly and added to by all those involved with the client. The development of these strategies requires several behaviours of the competent communicator. These are:

- Empathy.
- Perception and insight.
- Constant analysis of his/her own behaviours and those of the client.
- Taking particular account of behaviour which leads to particularly intense periods of interaction where the client is completely 'engaged' in the interaction.
- Recording and interpreting behaviours which invoke consistent responses from the client.
- Attempting to interpret consistent responses in a meaningful way.
- Recording of unsuccessful behaviours.

Records thus devised may be derived from behaviours observed by the speech and language therapist between client and carer, or between the speech and language therapist herself and the client. In the latter case video-recording is invaluable, enabling the therapist to analyse the communicative behaviours of the client and herself at a later stage.

Table 7.1 gives an account of the observations of strategies which a speech and language therapist may make to elicit responses with examples of possible behaviour by the client.

When observing which strategies trigger a communicative response from the client with profound intellectual and multiple disabilities it may also be useful to include information about factors in the environment which are conducive to successful interaction, and the effect of the introduction of toys or objects or other clients into the session.

It is also valuable to carry out a more traditional skills-based communication assessment to allow a more systematic analysis of communication strengths and deficits. Having observed the strategies which elicit a communicative response from a profoundly disabled client, the next stage is to observe the listening and visual skills of the client. Table 7.2 gives an account of the way in which listening skills can be observed with the client group.

Table 7.1 Observations of strategies which the care-giver or therapist may use to elicit a response from a client

Strategy	Client's response
Example 1	
Body proximity and position	
lying beside client	Client maintains fixed eye-gaze,
touching	smiles and vocalises using an open
facing each other	vowel sound
	Turntaking with C/T during vocalisation
Movements	
stroking client's face	Intense interaction maintained for 3 min with client very relaxed and absorbed
Facial expression	
smiling	
looking at client's face	
Vocalisation	
imitating client's vocalisations	
Example 2	
Body proximity and position	
sitting on floor, with client sitting astride C/T with head on C/T's shoulder	Rocking with C/T. When C/T stopped rocking, client rocked more vigorously until C/T began to rock again
Movement	
rocking backwards and forwards gently then stopping	Interaction maintained for several minutes with client cuddling into C/T and gradually reducing vigour of rocking response when C/T immediately responded each time
Facial expression	
unsmiling	
Vocalisation	
none	

C/T = Care-giver/Therapist.

Table 7.2 Ways in which listening skills may be used with clients with profound intellectual and multiple disabilities

Listening skills

Response to sound

Response to a sound outside the client's vision, e.g. rattle, bell or musical instrument:
    blinks
    startles

Table 7.2 contd.

stills
changes facial expression
turns to sound
reaches for object

Response to a familiar voice

Calling name; talking quietly; singing:
   blinks
   startles
   stills
   changes facial expression
   turns to sound

Visual skills

Eye contact

Ability to maintain eye contact:
   without therapist talking to client
   when therapist talks to client
   when therapist looks away does client attempt to acquire therapist's attention
and initiate eye contact?

Fixing on an object

Produce an interesting toy or brightly coloured object, e.g. Christmas tree decoration, tinsel, a torch:
   ignores object
   gazes, shares joint-attention of object with therapist
   gazes alternately at object and therapist
   reaches for object

Visual tracking

Ability to visually follow objects moving vertically or horizontally within client's field of vision, e.g. pull-along toy, ball (rolled or dropped), wind-up toy (monkey on a stick, clown on a ladder), bubbles:
   ignores object
   follows horizontal movement
   follows vertical movement

Having observed the effect of communicative strategies on the client's communicative behaviour and having observed the client's listening and visual skills, the speech and language therapist must then observe the pre-linguistic skills of the client. These are summarised in Table 7.3.

Table 7.3 Pre-linguistic skills of the client with profound intellectual and multiple disabilities

Anticipation

Does client demonstrate any anticipatory behaviours during familiar singing games and tickling games, e.g. *'Round and Round the Garden', 'This Little Piggy', 'Peek-a-Boo'*, knocking over a tower of bricks?

Reciprocity

Does client 'turntake' during:
    vocal imitation play (client vocalises; therapist vocalises)
    movement games, e.g. patting, stroking, rocking
    object exchange (therapist gives a toy or object to client who gives it back to therapist)?

Cause and effect

Is client able to understand toys or activities requiring knowledge of causality, e.g. knocking over a tower of bricks; operating a jack-in-a-box; operating switch toys or a computer switch?

Attention seeking

How does client respond when ignored?

Imitation

Does client imitate any patterns of vocalisation or movement?

Initiation

Does client initiate any interaction through vision, movement, vocalisation or touch?

Object permanence

Can client find a favourite object or toy when:
    partially hidden
    completely hidden?

Choice-making

Is client able to choose between two different kinds of food or drink or two objects or toys?
    no evidence of choice-making, passively accepts either of them
    will not accept either item
    inconsistently chooses item
    consistently chooses item

The fourth set of observations which the speech and language therapist must undertake relates to the observation of actual communicative
skills. Five areas of communicative skills are central to any such observations and these are enumerated in Table 7.4.

Table 7.4 Areas of communicative skills

Use of gesture

Does client use any idiosyncratic gestures which are interpreted by care-givers as
having meaning?

Communication of basic needs

What states does client communicate: pleasure/unhappiness/discomfort; pain;
hunger/thirst?

Any further basic needs which client is able to communicate, e.g. demanding a
favourite toy/object, asking for television/music to be turned on?

Rejection/negation

Does client reject food, drink, toys, activities or people? How does he do this?

Expressing desire for recurrence of objects/actions

Does client ask for objects/actions to be repeated? How does he do this?

Symbolic functioning

Present client with a variety of objects, e.g. cup, hairbrush, toothbrush, face flannel,
teddybear, doll, car. Is he able to use or play with these appropriately?

It is apparent that the assessment of clients with profound intellectual or multiple disabilities is a skilled and complex business. Extreme
sensitivity and insight are required and this can only be gained through
experience and knowledge of such people and through building a
close relationship with the particular individual being assessed. It is the
very foundations of communication that are being analysed.
Communication may consist of obvious motor movements, vocalisations or facial expressions or they may equally be manifested as subtle
changes in bodily posture or muscle tension. These communicative
attempts by the client may occur spontaneously, but often they will
occur only in response to a specific cue from the care-giver or therapist. If these communication foundations are to be developed, the
responses of the care-giver or therapist must be consistent and, in
order to achieve this, the therapist will use all her senses during assessment and subsequent therapy.

Many professionals are likely to be involved in working with the client with profound intellectual and multiple disabilities. The recent *Community Care Act* in the UK requires that multi-professional assessments are conducted in order to provide appropriate packages of care which cross traditional professional boundaries. In order to conduct such assessments effectively all professionals are being required to re-evaluate their role in a multi-disciplinary team and to identify their specific 'core skills' in order to eliminate duplication. It is important that there is neither duplication of actual assessment procedures nor of advice given to clients and their care-givers if confusion for the client is to be avoided.

The role of the speech and language therapist with these clients is to facilitate their development of communication by enabling the people who interact with them on a daily basis to communicate as successfully as possible. This approach of enabling the non-disabled people encourages as many 'quality' exchanges as possible. In order to do this, a therapist uses her core skills: those of observing and analysing the non-linguistic interlocutors and structuring this information in such a way that it can be understood and used by the non-disabled person to change communication strategies. Thus, care-givers and professionals enhance their communication skills and promote more effective communication with the disabled person.

References

Bates, E., Camaioni, L. and Volterra, V. (1975) The acquisition of performatives prior to speech. *Merrill-Palmer Quarterly* 21, 205–216

Brazelton, T.B., Koslowski, B. and Main, M. (1974) The origins of reciprocity: the early mother–infant interaction. In: Lewis, M. and Rosemblum, L.A. (eds). *The Effect of the Infant on its Caregiver*. New York: John Wiley

Bruner, J.S. (1977) Early social interaction and language acquisition. In: Schaffer, H.R. (Ed.). *Studies in Mother–Infant Interaction*. London: Academic Press

Burford, B. (1988) Action cycles: rhythmic actions for engagement in children and young adults with profound mental handicap. *European Journal of Special Needs Education* 3 (4), 189–206

Coupe, J., Barber, M. and Murphy, D. (1987) Affective communication. In: Coupe, J. and Goldbart, J. (eds). *Communication Before Speech*. London: Croom Helm

Dewart, H. and Summers, S. (1988) *The Pragmatics Profile of Early Communication Skills*. Windsor: NFER-Nelson

Evans, P. and Ware, J. (1987) *'Special Care' Provision: The Education of Children with Profound and Mental Learning Difficulties*. Windsor: NFER-Nelson

Kiernan, C. and Reid, B. (1987) *The Pre-Verbal Communication Schedule*. Windsor: NFER-Nelson

King, F. (1989) Assessment of pragmatic skills. *Child Language Teaching and Therapy* 5 (2), 191–201

Knight, C. (1991) Developing communication through interaction. In: Watson, J. (Ed.). *Innovatory Practice and Severe Learning Difficulties*. Edinburgh: Moray House Publications

Leeming, K., Swann, W., Coupe, J. and Mittler, P. (1979) *Teaching Language and Communication to the Mentally Handicapped*. London: Methuen Educational

Murphy, G. (1987) Direct observation as an assessment tool in functional analysis and treatment. In: Hogg, J. and Rayne, N. (eds). *Assessment in Mental Handicap*. London: Croom Helm

Newson, J. (1977) An intersubjectivity approach to the systematic study of mother–infant interaction. In: Schaffer, H.R. (Ed.). *Studies in Mother–Infant Interaction*. New York: Academic Press

Newson, J. (1979) The growth of shared understandings between infant and caregiver. In: Bullowa, M. (Ed.). *Before Speech: The Beginnings of Interpersonal Communication*. Cambridge University Press

Nind, M. and Hewett, D. (1988) Interaction as curriculum. *British Journal of Special Education* 15, 55–57

Pawlby, S.J. (1977) Imitative interaction. In: Schaffer, H.R. (Ed.). *Studies in Mother–Infant Interaction*. London: Academic Press

Schaffer, H.R. (1977) Early interactive development. In: Schaffer, H.R. (Ed.). *Studies in Mother–Infant Interaction*. London: Academic Press

Stern, D.N. (1977) The infant's stimulus world during social interaction. In: Schaffer, H.R. (Ed.). *Studies in Mother–Infant Interaction*. London: Academic Press

Trevarthon, C. (1979) Communication and co-operation in early infancy: a description of primary intersubjectivity. In: Bullowa, M. (Ed.). *Before Speech: The Beginnings of Interpersonal Communication*. Cambridge University Press

Watson, J. and Knight, C. (1991) An evaluation of intenstive interactive teaching with pupils with very severe learning difficulties. *Child Language Teaching and Therapy* 7 (3), 310–325

Chapter 8
Self-perception: the therapist in the process of change

Margaret Leahy

The focus of attention in this chapter is the therapist, not the client. Whereas this may be in contrast to the other chapters, it also complements them; the context of therapy is that of two people acting together to bring about change, and change in therapy is not limited to the client. By seeking help, the client shows a willingness to enter into a relationship with the therapist which will be of benefit and assistance in resolving a problem, or at least understanding it differently. The therapist also enters into the relationship with the welfare of the client as the stated primary concern but, hopefully, the relationship will also benefit the therapist. Since the focus here is questioning and discerning feelings, attitudes and issues concerned with the personal development of the therapist, it is natural to feel threatened initially, but this element of threat — if used creatively — may serve better to understand some of the difficulties a client experiences when exploring issues of a deeply personal nature. In a sense, the therapist may experience what it is like to be her own client and the reflexive nature of therapy may become more apparent.

Altruistic motives and interest in people may be assumed to be present to some degree when an individual chooses to become a therapist. But is this the overriding objective in therapy? What has a therapist to gain from therapy? And, has she anything to lose? Most people working in the so-called caring professions have a very good idea of what the client has to gain from therapy but, too often, the personal gains of the therapist from therapy are unquestioned. Certainly, the altruistic motive of practising therapy is well accepted and, in effect, is the foundation of the profession. But the importance given to this motivation may shift up and down depending on the work on hand. So why would it vary and what else can take precedence over it? In addressing questions such as these we are asking, ultimately, can therapy be therapeutic for the therapist?

The notion of self-actualisation

The therapist has to be sensitive to the needs of her client in a way that supersedes her own. But there is a case to be made for achieving a balance between one's own interests and those of the client. The humanistic point of view in psychology emphasises each person's expression of self as an individual within a social matrix which comprises many unique and individually different selves. Maslow (1968) described such expression as an impulse to improve oneself in actualising potential, thus moving in the direction of human fulfilment, a process he called 'self-actualisation'. He outlined a hierarchy of basic human needs arranged from the most potent to the least potent as follows:

1. Physiological needs (hunger and thirst).
2. Safety needs (security).
3. Love and belongingness needs (security and affection).
4. Esteem needs (affection and regard).
5. Self-actualisation needs (self-fulfilment).

Underlying this scheme is the assumption that lower-order, more potent needs must be at least somewhat satisfied before an individual can become aware of, or motivated by, higher-order needs, so the need for self-actualisation comes to the fore when the earlier needs are sufficiently satisfied. Working as a therapist may well serve some of the more basic needs, as well as the higher-order ones, and development may cease before the focus on self-actualisation.

Becoming the kind of person one wants to become and reaching the peak of one's potential is not achieved easily or automatically. Essentially, a therapist's personal development of the less potent — but arguably the most important — needs of esteem and self-actualisation may be thought to be egocentric. Dryden (1987) refers to this apparent egocentricity as 'enlightened self-interest' and considers it important that priority be given to one's own long-term goals in order to achieve happiness. This necessarily involves assuming a responsibility for one's own development as a therapist and as a person and examining personal awareness.

Personal awareness of the therapist

Although the individuality of the client is emphasised in therapy, the individuality of the therapist is undermined, probably because of professional stereotyping of what a 'good therapist' should be. The personal characteristics usually associated with the therapeutic role include warmth, acceptance of others, flexibility, creativity and objectivity, but the degree to which any one is important over the others (and over specialised knowledge) is not specified and, arguably, should never be specified, as each therapist has characteristic motives, strengths and weaknesses that are brought into play in different ways and at different times and influence therapy to a powerful extent. This contribution to the therapeutic process is an important variable in bringing about success, but it is not well researched and tends to be overshadowed by rigorous and prolonged student training in skills and techniques. Although such training under supervision functions to protect client interests, the development of the therapist's personality, style and individuality should not be neglected. If therapists are 'self-created' (Hayhow and Levy, 1989) then learning about the self is a major part of the process of becoming a more effective therapist, a process which continues throughout the therapist's working life. Havens (1986) refers to Matisse's exhortation to his students *'Go out and see a flower for the first time'*, i.e. to see without the usual baggage of presuppositions or expectations and assume an unbiased approach. Whereas this is a familiar approach used with clients (recognising that we can never be altogether unbiased), it is one we may fail to explore with the client's partner-in-practice, the therapist.

Few are formally prepared for the self-assessment and examination involved and, as mentioned, there may be elements of threat and uneasiness in beginning it. But the exploration is something of an adventure, one that can only help us in the process of *becoming* — a process that never ends. There are several possible starting points and the choice of any one will be dictated by the time on hand and previous experience. One that may be useful is the autobiography specifying important facts about oneself. McKay, Davis and Fanning (1983) suggest a number of headings which could be included, e.g. 'What school was like for you?', 'Your favourite teacher?', 'Your biggest loss?', 'Your most wonderful moment?', 'Your greatest achievement' and 'The funniest thing that ever happened to you'. Using this kind of information about oneself is similar to the first level of contact in a conversation: the information disclosed is not deep and not threatening, but it is revealing. McKay, Davies and Fanning (1983) then consider moving on to a deeper level of exploration involving thoughts, feelings and needs, e.g. considering a belief to which you are committed, a fear you once had, a concern for the future, problems in old relationships. In disclosing this level of information in conversation, there will be a deeper level of intimacy involved in the relationship; similarly, by specifying feelings and needs for yourself you will become more consciously aware of aspects of your 'real self'. Munro, Manthei and Small (1989) argue that such increased awareness of oneself and personal motivation will enable one to work more effectively with others. They suggest several useful self-examination exercises, one of which involves addressing the following issues.

As a therapist:

- I am becoming the kind of person who ...
- My strengths are ...
- My weaknesses are ...
- What I need most from people is ...
- What I give to people most of the time is ...

(It may be useful to question also, *'What pleases me most about doing therapy is ...'* and *'What disturbs me most about doing therapy is ....)*

The Character Sketch (Appendix A) (Kelly, 1955) is another exercise that helps to explore personal issues as if looking in from the outside. Writing the sketch in the third person encourages a certain detachment that allows the writer more freedom in expression. Hayhow and Levy (1989) suggest that two sketches be written, one of 'me as a person' and one of 'me as a therapist'. Satir (1978) follows a similar line of enquiry in discussing *Your Resource Wheel* (Appendix B), the various layers of which serve different functions and can temporarily stand alone but more usually interact and need the others to function fully.

Personal needs and motives may also be addressed directly by considering, for example, *'How much do I need to be helpful or nurturant?' 'How much do I need to be powerful and controlling?' 'How much do I need to be 'doing good'?' 'How much do I need people to be dependent on me?' 'How much do I need to be successful?' 'How important is it that clients like me?'.* It is important to remember that any or all of the above can be valid and essential at different stages in becoming a therapist.

Values, attitudes and biases of the therapist

Reviewing personal history will increase awareness of how family and experiences of a particular culture have shaped values and beliefs. Munro, Manthei and Small (1989) suggest the use of family photographs as an aid to recall in considering how the family operated and how it might still influence one's behaviour as a person and as a therapist. In a sense, this mirrors the procedure we use with clients to get to know about them and 'where they are coming from'. It is important to remember that personal values shape attitudes and biases and that these may remain relatively stable throughout life, regardless of how objective we feel we may have become. For example, it is well accepted that speech and language therapists hold a negative stereotype of 'the stutterer' (Horsley and Fitzgibbon, 1987; Woods and Williams, 1976). As a fluency clinician of almost 20 years' standing, aware of that negative stereotype, the author believed that she did not have negative attitudes towards the person who stutters but a recent experience proved otherwise.Going to meet a newly referred client in the waiting area the author found the people there were relaxed, smiling and chatting quietly and immediately thought that her client was not among them. Wrong! Despite having a moderately severe stutter, the client in question was not tense, anxious, unwilling to interact with strangers or unfriendly, as she had unconsciously anticipated. Experiences such as this serve to underline the fact that unawareness and conscious denying of attitudes and biases does not negate them.

It may be interesting to examine some personal attitudes and biases. Commonly held stereotypes are those associated with names, appearance, race, religion and social class. Consider, for example, what characteristics come to mind when some names are mentioned (alternatively, consider how would you be different if you — or someone you know — were called by a different name, e.g. *Angela, Rupert, Zara, Gilbert, Mathilda*, or *Abernathy Smith, Thomas-Davis, Finkelstein, Murphy, Obutu*, or *Butler*.

What other characteristics come to mind when someone is described as any of the following: tall; thin; slim; fat; long-haired male; long-haired blond female. (Again, how would you be different if you were, for example, tall, thin?)

Client categories may also be addressed: the person who stutters; the adult with aphasia, dysarthria, dyspraxia; the child with language disorder; the adult with laryngectomy, voice disorder, etc.

The therapeutic relationship

Therapy has been described as a *pas de deux* (Casement, 1985) where both therapist and client play an important part, which is interdependent in different ways for both parties: the reflexiveness mentioned earlier. This mutual influence is part of the successful therapeutic relationship which Kelly (1958) compares to embarking on a sea voyage 'as shipmates on the very same adventure' (p. 232). This analogy conjures up a picture of cooperation and mutual respect which emphasises equality between the two people who have different expertise: the therapist is expert in specialist knowledge and approaches to alleviating the problem directly or indirectly; the client is expert in his knowledge and experience of his problem, which is unique to him. The therapist's acknowledgment of this understanding and the client's wish to change and to deal with the inherent risks involved, allows for a collaboration between experts so that therapy becomes more of a partnership than a transfer of information or expertise.

The 'adventure' that is therapy for Kelly (1958) is construed differently according to the model the therapist uses in working with clients. It follows that the nature of the client–therapist relationship will be different as it depends on the understanding the therapist has of how behaviour may be changed. Speech and language therapists generally have tended to use traditional medical and behaviourist models that have influenced ways of understanding behaviour for many years, the most prominent of which are outlined here.

Models of intervention

Three common models of intervention have been used in speech and language therapy: the medical, the behavioural and the facilitative model.

Medical model

The medical model follows the so-called 'hard sciences', stressing empiricism. Here, the process of diagnosis is a dominant feature derived from observing signs and symptoms that are presented. Pathology, the branch of medicine that pertains to the origins, nature and development of changes in the physiology that determine the disease, is linked with the symptoms and the aetiology or causal factors are evaluated. This logical series of steps provides the rational basis for treatment and understanding aetiology is the basis of preventive therapy (Kahn and Earle, 1982).

Although there are several justifications for classifying disorders of speech and language in accordance with physiological and anatomical changes (i.e. where the aetiology is observable and known) and establishing treatment on that basis, there are also many instances where aetiology is unknown and bears little or no relation to focus of therapy.

Behavioural model

Behaviourism developed during the early years of the twentieth century, at around the same time that the profession of speech and language therapy was developing. In its most radical form, behaviourism sees human actions as derived solely from two sources: biological deprivation and the individual's learning history. In influencing change and learning, the concepts of motivation and reward are central and input is directly linked to output. In such a theory, there is no place for the concepts of mind and free will (Nelson-Jones, 1982). Behaviourism stresses empiricism in its methods and the active role is performed by the therapist who analyses the problem, determines the behaviour of the (passive) client to be shaped and changed and proceeds to do so. Throughout the process there is a commitment to objectivity in the analysis and treatment of the problem, with detailed and precise specification of aims and techniques. Again, adherence to empiricism attracts therapists who may feel vulnerable because of criticism levelled at the profession about being a 'quasi-science' (see also Siegal, 1987) or not a science at all. The pervasiveness of the behaviourist model is evident where motivation and reward are considered the major determining factors of successful outcome in therapy.

Facilitative models

In facilitative models of intervention the values, perceptions, experiences and understanding of the client take precedence over those of the therapist in determining and working with the problem for which the client has sought help. The major questions therapy poses are *'How is the client experiencing the problem?'* and *'How may this be changed?'* as opposed to *'What are the symptoms, severity and aetiology of the disorder?'* and *'How may I change these?'*. Essentially, the client directs the therapist as to how to treat him (Keeney, 1983). Decisions taken in therapy are the responsibility of both client and therapist, with the client taking the dominant role. Whereas there are many theories that fit the facilitative model, Kelly's personal construct theory is the one most widely used in speech and language therapy since Fransella (1972) applied it in working with stuttering. Kelly considered the person as scientist, continually forming, testing and revising hypotheses about oneself, one's behaviour and one's world. The construing of similarities and differences in events allows us to build up a system of constructs which are, in effect, our experience of reality. The process of construing is one that is subject to change according to changing experiences and behaviour is understood as 'the experiment', where we test our hypothesis, formulated on the basis of previous experience.

This understanding of behaviour is different from the two models mentioned already: the medical model (*'You are a victim of your biology'*) and the behavioural (*'You are a victim of your reinforcement schedule'*), where behaviour change is seen as the main responsibility of the expert therapist with the client playing a more passive, non-expert role. The major decisions are left in the hands of the expert and the non-expert cooperates and follows advice. Despite the recognition that scientific knowledge is 'of its nature provisional and permanently so' (Popper, in Magee, 1973, p. 26), the expert role confers on the therapist a kind of omnipotence and certain knowledge which may lead her to assume such knowledge and substitute terms, such as 'multiple coexisting factors' for *'I don't know'* in addressing clients' questions.

Along with equality and cooperation between the two parties involved in the therapy enterprise, uncertainty and openness are characteristic of personal construct work. Instead of decreasing the scientific nature of the work, uncertainty — when used creatively — increases it, and openness generates understanding. Knowledge changes and grows through raising questions, formulating hypotheses and experimenting. Unless we question accepted facts, consider alternatives and test them, our knowledge stagnates.

Evaluating your theory

When we work as therapists we follow guiding principles that underlie our approach and organisation. These guiding principles or theories are often more implicit than explicit and we may be unaware of them. But — as with attitudes — a lack of awareness or difficulty in specifying them, does not mean they do not exist. Becoming more aware of guiding principles will increase understanding of the process of change and perhaps lead to reviewing and renewing that understanding. If you favour one theory in particular, does it provide a broad enough base for working with diverse clients? Or do you change theories when working with clients presenting with different problems? Addressing the following questions may be useful for elucidating your theory of change:

- What is your belief about how people change?
- What does this approach stress and why does it appeal to you?
- Where did you acquire this theory?
- How does this theory affect your own lifestyle, experiences and values?
- How do you see your own life experiences as influencing your therapy style?

Hayhow and Levy (1989) suggest exploring how a number of activities (e.g. reading a novel, talking to a close friend, planning games for a children's party, etc.) are similar or different from therapy. Having listed the constructs associated with therapy, mark the preferred pole of each from your point of view as a therapist and note any incompatibilities. Increasing awareness of how you experience therapy in this way may lead you to change your way of working and open further avenues for exploration.

Personal change

If you think you are not functioning as you would prefer — either personally and/or professionally — it may be useful to highlight those areas and consider personal change. In doing this, issues which need to be clarified include: if changing any, which would be easy and which difficult to change? List your options and consider the advantages of each option. Decide your course of action and begin to experiment with change.

Experiencing personal change is arguably the best way of discovering how discomforting change can be and it will help us to understand the kinds of difficulties that clients experience when we expect them to change in therapy. Choose a personal behaviour that you would like to change. What are the implications of making this change? Tschudi's (1977) *ABC* technique is one way of exploring this: A = present behaviour; A2 = desired behaviour; B = disadvantages of present behaviour; B2 = disadvantages of desired behaviour; C = advantages of present behaviour; C2 = advantages of desired behaviour. For example, *'I want to become more fit'*.

A = I am not fit

A2 = I am fit

B = lack of energy, body in poor condition, a bit depressed

B2 = time-consuming effort, gear and club costs, sustained effort needed

C = no effort involved, time absorbed, no money, expended

C2 = I will feel better, look better work better and enjoy life more!

So expending time, money and effort and sustaining that expenditure are the costs of (and the obstacles to) changing the behaviour. This involves a re-organisation of schedules and priorities and the chances are that it will be difficult. Although this understanding may help in clearing a pathway to change, actual change only occurs if we begin to *do* something differently, i.e. experiment with change.

Experimenting with change

Kelly (1970) viewed behaviour as our principal means of enquiry. Behaviour follows a prediction or anticipation of the outcome of an event. Through our behaviour we commit ourselves to our enquiry about some matter and then we collect the evidence and review how well the prediction fitted. Take as a further example, deciding to change one's role in an unpleasant relationship. The behaviours that are the focus here could be, e.g. initiating conversation in a pleasant and personal manner. The prediction is that the outcome will be favourable, with the other person responding in a somewhat surprised but accepting manner, resulting in more easygoing interaction. The behaviour is to begin conversation by complimenting the other person on their appearance or on work well done. Difficulties anticipated might include, e.g. being sincere in the interaction and finding the appropriate compliment. If the outcome is positive as one predicted, this experiment will be repeated with the result that the relationship would become more pleasant. The actual performance of the new behaviour may be quite discomforting, however, in that one is placing oneself in unfamiliar circumstances and experiencing the threats of this unfamiliarity.

The internal supervisor

Using the skills, insights and questions of the supervisor may also improve one's understanding. Hayhow and Levy (1989) recommend that supervision be regarded as necessary for the therapist's personal growth and development. They suggest that it become part of the therapist's normal working hours and that it focuses not only on the client but also on the therapist's personal threats and areas of anxiety. Such continuing supervision or detailed discussion with a supportive co-therapist — either of which would be ideal — may not always be available, but developing one's own internal supervisor (Casement, 1985) may be an excellent alternative. This would involve scheduling a specified time and organising it to consider personal ideas, feelings and behaviours as a therapist. As a beginning therapist, the supervisor functions by providing a form of control and support that makes it safe for the student to become engaged in therapy. Through questioning and discussion, understanding and insight regarding the client and oneself as a therapist are developed. Gradually, the student therapist acquires the capacity for reflection within the session and learns to monitor herself as well as the client: the internal supervision has begun and it continues as one develops in the process of becoming a better therapist, a process that is never completed. Development of self-awareness will have some negative implications but usually it is a useful and positive process.

Casement (1985) refers to the spiral experienced by supervisors of student therapists:

> ... they are back where they have been before (the beginning of training or the beginning of a treatment), but also where they have never been before (p. 33).

He also points out the endless opportunities that supervisors have to re-examine their own work when looking closely at the work of students. It is in this same re-examining process that the internal supervisor engages.

Risks in therapy interaction

Relationships generally begin with conversations and, as with any conversation, there are elements of risk involved. Wardhaugh (1985) mentions some of these, including the risk of being hurt or of inflicting hurt; the risk of being criticised or of criticising; the risk of being complimented and having to accept it and live up to it; the risk that the other person's sincerity is suspect, assuming of course that one's own is not. In the clinic there may be other risks as well. The client has to speak and generally this is not something that comes easily, otherwise he would not be there. He has to disclose intimate data about himself and his problem, that he would normally not disclose to a stranger. Some of this may be shocking or upsetting so there is a risk of being rejected. Some may appear irrelevant to the client, so there is a risk of appearing uncooperative and perhaps rejecting of the therapist if all is not revealed.

The therapist shares some of these risks and runs some others. It is the therapist who carries the responsibility to initiate rapport and thereby set the scene for all that follows. If this proves difficult or unsatisfactory, the client may not return. Acting as a professional, the therapist is cast in a role that demands several qualities and skills *inter alia*, empathy, specialist knowledge and an ability to communicate easily. If any of these appear suspect then the enterprise may be doomed, so not only would she lose face professionally, but the meaningfulness of her role as therapist is called into question.

The therapist is responsible for involving the client in therapy and ensuring a clear understanding of the roles of therapist and client, the process of therapy and the means whereby individual expectations may be met. Some of the most important considerations are language issues, self-disclosure, empathy and objectivity.

The language of the therapist

The initial responsibilities of the therapist are to establish rapport, take a case history and provide an overview of therapy. Depending on the model of therapy chosen, this can be either a one-way system or more of an exchange of ideas and information. Taking a case history may involve a series of questions in a clear subject–object differentiation where *I*, the therapist, question *You*, the client, (so that *'I can understand the symptoms that define the problem and determine the treatment'*). Generally, questions asked in this approach are closed and limiting, seeking specific information that the therapist wants.

Alternatively the session may begin with the therapist fostering an alliance with the client in explaining the particular approach taken, e.g. *'We're here to work together and to do that we have to find out more about each other'*. Or, the direction of the questions/answers can be left up to the client after an opening *'What brings you here today?'*. Use of open questions allows the client to reply in a way that suits him, putting him in control of the information provided, but use of the term 'problem' when first meeting clients, even in open-ended questions may signify that the professional's interest is only in the client's weaknesses (Cunningham and Davis, 1985). Later in therapy, when movement has begun and the roles played by therapist and client are clearly defined, the author has found it useful to begin sessions with *'What can I do for you to-day?'*, although Cunningham and Davis (1985) advise that it may wrongly imply that the responsibility for action is with the professional and not the client.

Empathy

The concept of empathy with clients is stressed as important by all therapists. Empathy involves a kind of sensitivity to the client that indicates that the therapist understands the meaning of the client's particular experience. Dryden (1987) suggests two kinds of empathy: affective and philosophic, where both feelings and the philosophy that underlies those feelings are understood. As well as establishing basic conditions in therapy, Gregory (1978) considers it important to be empathetic because it serves to initiate in the client a process of self-evaluation. It also serves in the development of a trusting, open and respectful relationship.

It is vital not just to be empathetic, but to be able to communicate this precisely, clearly and accurately by reflecting meaning back to the client. This is not done so much by saying *'I know how you feel'* or *'I understand'* as by stating one's own interpretation of the feeling expressed (Cunningham and Davis, 1985). Havens (1986) differentiates between *simple* and *complex empathetic statements*. In the first instance, indicating attention and understanding through non-verbal expressions, e.g. nodding, frowning and smiling at appropriate times, shows minimal empathy. The use of unaccented adjectives such as 'awful' and 'wonderful' may express emotional attentiveness, whereas accented exclamations may seem patronising.

Complex empathetic statements reflect a deeper understanding of what the client is expressing, e.g. *'No one understands'* suggests that the therapist understands that no one understands and invites the reflection that some one should have understood. Havens (1986) also uses personal pronouns in statements with 'no wonder' or 'it is natural' to express that the event and feeling are joined and reconnected. So *'No wonder you were frightened'* (pp 55–58) places the therapist where the client was. Similarly, Cunningham and Davis (1985) provide examples, such as *'You feel you are not as capable as you should be'* to the mother who states, *'She keeps crying, no matter what I do ...'* and *'You were prepared to suffer this indignity ...'* (p. 101) to the mother who continued to seek help for her son in the face of professionals' rejection of his need for therapy.

It should be recognised that mastery of language alone does not constitute empathy. As Havens (1986) points out:

> A therapist's disinterest, inattentiveness, or lack of ability to contain the other's feelings can alter the effectiveness of even the most appropriate language. On the other hand, a powerful ability can redeem language that is otherwise prying or even critical (p. 53).

The language of objectivity

Whereas the language of empathy generates trust and a kind of closeness between therapist and client, it is balanced by the use of language, of objectivity (and perhaps other codes: see Leahy, 1989) which helps to establish and maintain professional distance. Although equality in the relationship is encouraged, it has to be recognised that it is not enough for supplying some needs, and formality and tradition can act as protection for clients (Kahn and Earle, 1982). The language of objectivity describes facts, gives information and it may be used subjectively to express opinions. Reviewing the facts about a disorder, outlining procedures to be used and describing responsibilities in therapy are all done using the language of objectivity.

Self-disclosure

Self-disclosure occurs at several different levels, e.g. through dress, body language, voice and intonation. Messages are sent and received, both intentionally and unintentionally, in all relationships. Despite a desire to be approved by a client and a desire to develop openness in the therapy relationship, verbal self-disclosure on the part of the therapist may not always be appropriate. Disclosing limited personal details to the client at the beginning of therapy may help to establish the relationship, but lengthy stories or personal anecdotes during the course of therapy serve to shift the focus from the client and may even be considered unethical, in that it may be serving the needs of the therapist rather than those of the client (Van Hoose and Kottler, 1985). Appropriate disclosure where the therapist expresses feelings that relate directly to the client's experiences, may help increase understanding. Such disclosure allows the therapist to be herself in serving the needs of the client.

The process of examining self-awareness is integral to the development of the practice of therapy. The contribution of the therapist in therapy is powerful and unique in a similar way to that of the client. Therapy is a shared experience, a partnership that by its nature necessarily centres on the client, but not exclusively so, as has been demonstrated here.

Recognising limits

Although speech and language therapists will be qualified to work with the entire range of clients presenting with diverse speech and language problems, most will find themselves with a preference for working within particular disorder groups or perhaps age groups. Some may even find that they prefer to work more in management or administration, or in the academic world with a limited amount of contact with clients. Whatever the preferences, it takes wisdom and courage to admit that you cannot work effectively with everyone and, more importantly, that you do not *have* to work effectively with everyone. Likes and dislikes, biases and negative attitudes have to be realised and confronted. Some may change, some may not. The responsibility for effectiveness in therapy is not exclusively that of the therapist. The client and his family share in it, the team shares in it, the administration shares in it, and the social values of the community share in it (as realised by funding and action). Developing awareness of the self and recognising your place in the matrix of society within the larger system that is the human race and the smaller systems that are the immediate family and the working place, will help put things in perspective.

Appendix A

The Character Sketch

Instructions: "I want you to write a character sketch of (e.g. Harry Brown), just as if he were the principal character in a play. Write it as it might be written by a friend who knew him very intimately and very sympathetically, perhaps better than anyone could ever really know him. Be sure to write it in the third person. For example, start out by saying 'Harry Brown is ...'" (Kelly, 1955).

Appendix B

Virginia Satir's (1978) Resource Wheel

Satir (1978) describes the *resource wheel* in terms of layers, the first of which is the self — the 'I'. Around the 'I' is the body, the physiology which she describes as 'your house' and around which is the mind, the 'captain of your ship', which analyses what you see and hear. Around this layer are the emotions — your 'juice'. The senses make up the next layer in which input from the outside comes in and through which messages go out. The following layer is the communication layer, focusing on the 'I–thou' relationships and how they influence health, feelings and uses of the self. The centre of all is the soul or the 'life force' or essence which may or may not have a connection with organised religion. All of the layers occur within a context made up of time, space, light, air, water, colour, weather and season. All the layers are present and have life and are also interacting and continually moving — thoughts, feelings, body, senses, relationships. Discovering how these parts interact lets us know how we are treating ourselves and others.

References

Casement, P. (1985) *On Learning from the Patient*. London: Routledge

Cunningham, C. and Davis, H.D. (1985) *Working with Parents: Frameworks for Collaboration*. Milton Keynes: Open University Press

Dryden, W. (1987) *Counselling Individuals: the Rational–Emotive Approach*. London: Taylor & Francis

Fransella, F. (1972) *Personal Change and Reconstruction*. London: Academic Press

Gregory, H.H. (1978) The clinician's attitudes in counselling stutterer's speech. *Foundations of America* 18. Memphis

Havens, L. (1986) *Making a Contact*. Cambridge, MA: Harvard University Press

Hayhow, R. and Levy, C. (1989) *Working with Stuttering*. Bicester: Winslow Press

Horsley, I. and FitzGibbon, C.T. (1987) Stuttering children: investigation of a stereotype. *British Journal of Disorders of Communication* 22 (1), 19–36

Kahn, J. and Earle, E. (1982) *The Cry for Help and the Professional Response*. London: Pergamon

Keeney, B. (1963) *The Aesthetics of Change*. New York: Guildford Press

Kelly, G.A. (1955) *The Psychology of Personal Constructs*. New York: Norton

Kelly, G.A. (1958) Personal construct theory and the psychotherapeutic interview. In: Mather, B. (Ed.). *Clinical Psychology and Personality: The Selected Papers of George Kelly*. Huntington, NY: Krieger (1979)

Kelly, G.A. (1970) Behaviour is the experiment. In: Bannister, D. (Ed.). *Perspectives in Personal Construct Theory*. London: Academic Press

Leahy, M.M. (1989) Philosophy in intervention. In: Leahy, M.M. (Ed.). *Disorders of Communication: The Science of Intervention*. London: Whurr

Magee, B. (1973) Popper. London: Fontana

Maslow, A. (1968) *Towards a Psychology of Being*. New York: Van Rostrand Reinhold

McKay, M., Davis, M. and Fanning, P. (1989) *Messages: The Communication Book*. Oakland, CA: New Harbinger Publications

Munro, A., Manthei, B. and Small, J. (1989) *Counselling: The Skills of Problem-Solving*. London: Routledge

Nelson-Jones, R. (1982) *The Theory and Practice of Counselling Psychology*. London: Holt, Rinehart and Winston

Satir, V. (1978) *Your Many Faces*. Berkeley, CA: Celestial Arts

Siegal, G.M. (1987) The limits of science in communication disorders. *Journal of Speech and Hearing Disorders* 306

Tschudi, F. (1977) Loaded and honest questions. In: *New Perspectives in Personal Construct Theory*. London: Academic Press

Van Hoose, W.H. and Kottler, J.A. (1985) *Ethical and Legal Issues in Counseling and Psychotherapy*. San Francisco: Jossey-Bass

Woods, C.L. and Williams, D.E. (1976) Traits attributed to stuttering and normally fluent males. *Journal of Speech and Hearing Research* 19, 267–278

Subject Index

Author Index